The Food Doctor In the City

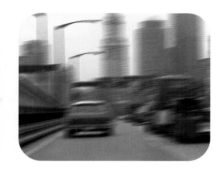

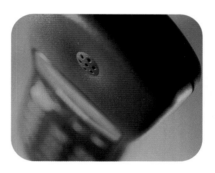

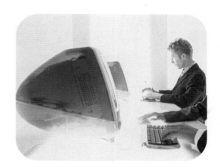

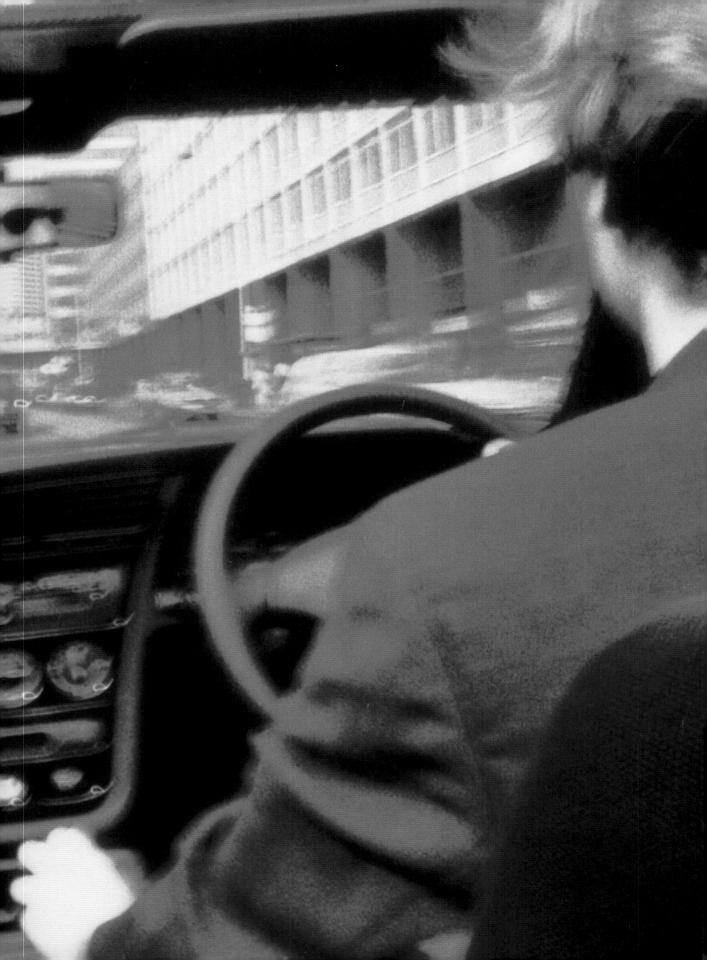

The Food Doctor In the City

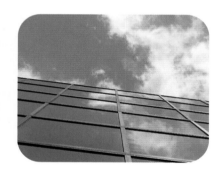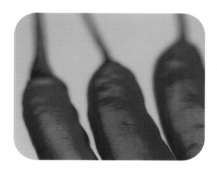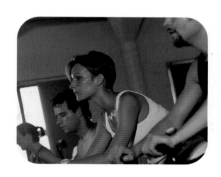

Maximum Health for Urban Living

Ian Marber Dip ION

www.thefooddoctor.com

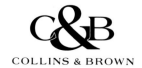

COLLINS & BROWN

For my mother and father, with love and thanks for their friendship, support, wit and wisdom.

I would like to thank the following colleagues and friends for their contributions and help: Juliet Alexander, Stefan Behmer, Simon Carey, Michael da Costa, Liz Dean, Betty Edelstein, Vicki Edgson, Fiona Gale, Mandy Greenfield, John Hadity, Andy Hockley, Chistopher Lloyd, Jani Phillips, Sonia Pugh, Rebecca Read, Bev Speight, Mary Thomas, Claire Wedderburn-Maxwell, Nigel Wright and Colin Ziegler.

First published in Great Britain in 2000
by Collins & Brown Limited
London House
Great Eastern Wharf
Parkgate Road
London SW11 4NQ

Distributed in the United States and Canada by Sterling Publishing Co.
387 Park Avenue South, New York, NY 10016 USA

3 5 7 9 8 6 4 2

British Library Cataloguing-in-Publication Data:
A catalogue record for this book is available from the British Library.

ISBN 1 85585 776 6

Designed by XAB
Edited by Mandy Greenfield

Reproduction by Global Colour, Malaysia
Printed and bound in Spain by Bookprint, S.L, Barcelona

SAFETY NOTE
The information in this book is not intended as a substitute for medical advice. Any person suffering from conditions requiring medical attention, or who has symptoms that concern them, should consult a qualified medical practictioner.

contents

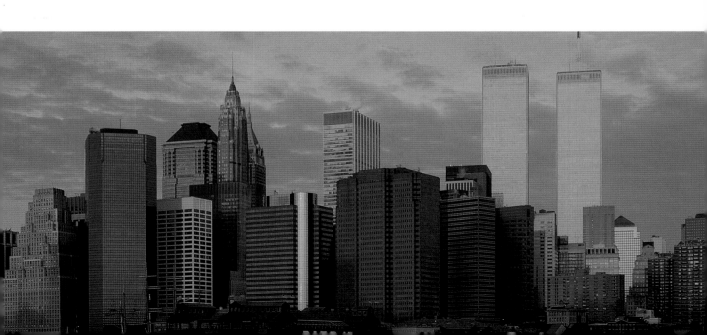

how to use
this book

This book is designed for those of us who choose to live in the city. It covers not just food and nutrition, but lifestyle and general health as well. While there is no typical city dweller, many urbanites have similar experiences and are potentially at greater risk from stresses and pollution than those who live in rural areas.

Furthermore, they are more likely to suffer from fatigue, 'lows' during the day, lack of energy, depression and anxiety, headaches, digestive disorders, immune-challenging situations and inflammatory ailments.

While we all know what we *should* be eating, many of us do not eat in such a way as to maximize our health, given both the challenges and the opportunities that city life can offer.

Eating optimally to increase your energy is easier than most of us might think.

The Food Doctor in the City shows you exactly what is best for you – from simple foods and nutrients to lifestyle plans, which you can adapt to fit the way you live your life. It has been designed to enable you either to make some simple changes or to rethink the whole way you eat and live, so that you can enjoy the best that your city has to offer. For example, do you feel tired in the afternoons, yet get a 'second wind' around 5 p.m.? Do you experience headaches often, or find that you have a bloated stomach by the end of the day? *The Food Doctor in the City* has the answers to these questions, and many more.

The book is divided into three parts. **Part One** examines the toxins, stresses and risks of city life, and investigates how the modern urban lifestyle affects bodies that were not designed for such consistent pressure. It looks at the process of detoxification, and at those foods that aid – or hinder – it.

The working environment is also covered, as the modern workplace can be stressful. We look at air quality, how it can affect your health (both indoors and out) and how best to redress the balance using foods found in every supermarket and café in town. And we hear so much these days about the potential risk posed by the frequent use of mobile telephones, but what is the truth behind this? *The Food Doctor in the City* shows you how best to eat for health so that the risk from low-level radiation from telephones and computer screens is minimized. Travelling in the city is another source of stress, but practical snack suggestions can help you avoid hunger and energy lows when you are on the go all day, without having to resort to boosts from caffeine and sugar.

Part Two explains how the City Plan, designed to help you survive a week in the city, fits into your daily life. Covering essential nutritional issues such as blood-sugar management (how best to combine protein, fibre and carbohydrates to feel vital and alert), the plan shows you what – and when – to eat during the day and before going out in the evening, how to improve your looks and how to exercise for maximum benefit. It reveals how you can find peace in the city and relax, get the sleep you need and counter anxiety, stress and depression with simple nutritional remedies. With tips on business lunches, deli snacks and the top-ten evening snacks and dinners, 'A Week in the City' will guide you successfully through the stresses of urban living.

Part Three shows you how to put the City Plan into action, with easy-to-make soups and starters, main courses, vegetable and grain recipes, fast lunches, plus delicious smoothies, all designed for the casual cook and the beginner alike. Advice on what food to choose when eating out in restaurants, plus different eating regimes to help boost your energy levels, and to calm and soothe you, covers all eventualities. With a detailed schedule revealing how best to manage a weekend detoxification plan, plus a Monday-to-Friday weight-management plan, **Part Three** shows you exactly what to do to achieve the best possible health in the city and how to thrive in an urban environment.

You can also visit the website at www.thefooddoctor.com.

1

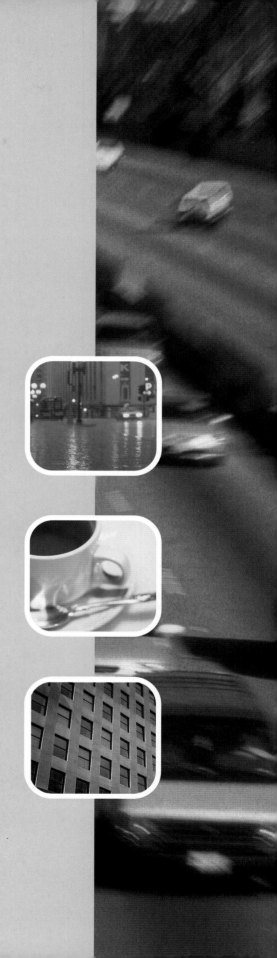

city
challenges

specific stresses

City life can bring with it specific situations and stresses, some of which we may be aware of and some of which occur internally. While we may get a buzz from the excitement and energy that we experience in the city, many seemingly innocuous situations can have negative long-term effects on the way we feel, both emotionally and physically.

The 'fight or flight' response

We are all conversant with stress, and our bodies were designed to handle and respond to stress in a positive manner, but the response was intended to be a short-term one. Our hunter-gatherer ancestors experienced stress in dangerous situations – perhaps while finding food. In response to perceived danger, the pituitary gland at the base of the skull stimulates the adrenal glands by the kidneys to release the hormone adrenaline, which in the short term has a positive effect as it prepares the body for action – originally for 'fight or flight'.

The level of stress that we experience every day in the city far exceeds that which we were designed for.

Modern life, however, rarely allows stress to be short-term, and many of us lead our lives in a state of constant stress. This does not just imply an external danger or threat – the body may also respond to internal stresses, such as disease, injury, anxiety or toxins.

In the city we are all used to standing in queues – be it at the train station, the bank or the coffee shop. Do you find yourself becoming easily irritated by such queues, because you are in a hurry to get back to work or to get home? In such a situation it is likely that your adrenal glands will produce adrenaline and your blood pressure will rise, which has various influences on the body. For instance, the muscles and the liver will release glucose from its stored form, glycogen, while internal energy is diverted away from your digestive system to your brain and muscles. See the chart on p. 12 on the effects of stress for a full explanation of how frequent adrenaline release can affect long-term health.

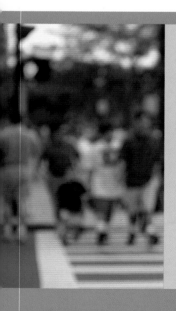

City stresses

Here are examples of the particular pressures that city life offers:

Lack of time to shop or eat	**Pollution**
Being away from home all day	**Drugs (both prescription and**
Exposure to viruses and bugs	**'street' drugs)**
Queues	**Traffic**
Commuting (including by car and public	**Smoking and smoky atmospheres**
transport)	**Lack of fresh air**
Lack of sunlight	**Pressurized work environments**
Social pressures	**Constant presence of other people**

Such external stresses will be familiar to almost everyone, but how aware are we of the way in which they can be detrimental to our health?

Internal stresses

Internal stresses, which we may not be aware of, also have a direct influence on how we function. For example, any nutrient deficiency can cause a potential problem internally. Drinking caffeinated drinks all day, like tea, coffee or sodas, can knock out vital minerals such as magnesium – an essential nutrient in combating stress, since the adrenal glands require adequate amounts of magnesium in order to function optimally.

The regular consumption of processed or 'fast' foods, which some people view as the easiest way to eat, given the pressures of city life, can further deplete essential nutrients, or place an unnecessary burden on body organs. Many of these foods contain excessive amounts of sugar and salt.

Most of us consume unnecessary salt in our diets (up to ten times as much as we actually need), and the addition of salt-laden foods can upset the normal rhythm of the heart or interrupt the natural flow of nutrients into and out of the body's cells. Salt affects us at a cellular level by having a negative affect on the sodium/potassium pump, which is responsible for the entry of nutrients into, and the removal of waste products from, the cell. In the long term this can reduce the cells' ability to function optimally.

Free radicals versus antioxidants

Let's look at another example: city life brings with it increased exposure to free radicals – very short-lived, destructive molecules made by the body – which have many damaging effects. They can impair the lining of the arteries, lead to internal inflammation or even to signs of ageing. While free radicals are a natural by-product of metabolism, their number is increased in city life by pollution, chemicals and stress.

The body has natural defences to protect it from free radicals, known as antioxidant compounds, but these rely on a sufficient amount of certain vitamins and minerals for their manufacture. These include vitamins A, C and E, in addition to the minerals selenium and zinc (and there are many others as well), so it is vital to eat sufficient of these nutrients to enable the body to make ample antioxidant compounds needed to counteract the free radicals. You can read more about free radicals and antioxidants on p. 18.

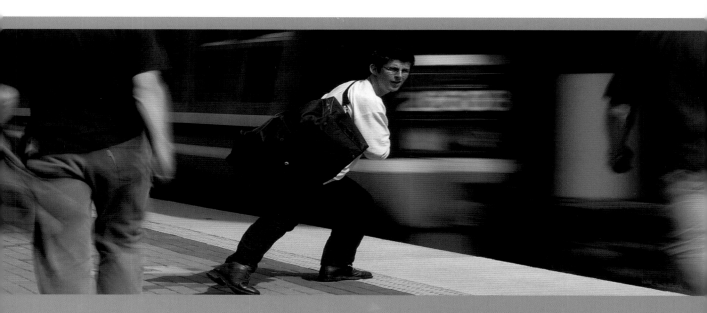

The effects of stress

SHORT-TERM	LONG-TERM
Amino acids are released from the muscles and bones to provide short-term energy.	The muscles and bone break down, without being replaced adequately.
Stored glucose, in the form of glycogen, is broken down releasing glucose into the blood for short-term energy.	The natural blood glucose balance is disrupted, leading to pressure on the adrenal glands and the pancreas.
Sodium is retained by the blood in order to raise blood pressure temporarily, so that nutrients and oxygen can be delivered more efficiently to the muscles, and waste and carbon dioxide can be removed.	Elevated blood pressure stresses the heart muscle; increased sodium levels interfere with the flow of nutrients into and out of the cells, as well as disturbing the natural rhythm of the heart.
Infection is resisted through the effects of cortisol, a steroid hormone that is raised at times of stress.	Risk of infection increases, as long-term raised cortisol production suppresses certain aspects of the immune response.
The raised levels of cortisol counter possible inflammation that might occur through injury.	Cortisol raises blood glucose levels, which triggers the release of the hormone insulin. Long-term stress can lead to exhaustion and the failure of insulin-producing cells.
Fats are released from the tissues for energy production to meet the body's extra requirements. This can, in some cases, increase cholesterol and blood lipid levels.	Raised fats in the blood lead to raised levels of triglycerides, which may increase the risk of cardiovascular disease.

what are toxins?

The word toxin (from the Latin *toxicum*) means poison. We are subjected to any number of potential toxins every day, in the air we breathe, the water we drink and the food we eat.

The liver is responsible for neutralizing these toxins by extracting the poisonous elements, then combining them with innocuous, naturally produced substances. This is done in two stages – in stage one the toxins may become more toxic as they are broken down, before being passed to the second stage, where the detoxification process is finished. In short, toxins enter the liver, where they are broken down by various chemical reactions into 'intermediate metabolites' (which act in a similar way to free radicals), then combined into the end-product, known as 'excretory derivatives'.

The final stage is excretion – toxins are eliminated from the body via the kidneys, the bowels or the skin. Many people who undertake a detoxification programme will experience some skin problems, highlighting the skin's role as a route of elimination.

If the liver, kidneys or bowel are working below par, due to pressure or stress, then the effective removal of toxins is compromised.

Toxins in the body

Toxins in the body are stored in the cells. They deplete the ability of the cells to function. Every cell in the body produces energy, and toxins stored at cellular level can hinder this process. In this way, toxins can potentially affect our energy levels.

Toxins can also pass through the protective layer of the brain, known as the blood-brain barrier. In normal circumstances this barrier serves to protect the brain from unwanted substances. However, many toxins have the ability to cross this layer and lodge in the brain

Potential pollutants and toxins

AIRBORNE POLLUTANTS
Pollen
Chemicals – household or industrial
Lead
Carbon monoxide
Cigarette smoke
CFCs (chlorofluorocarbons, found in aerosols, refrigerators, etc.)
Free radicals

FOOD AND WATER TOXINS
Chemicals/pesticides
Colourants
Aluminium
Chlorine
Bacteria

cells. The best example is mercury, to which many of us are vulnerable. Mercury in the brain can affect cognitive function and also our mood and self-perception (see p. 16).

For those of us who are unaffected by mercury, there are other toxins that can also cross the blood-brain barrier. Yeasts and microbes, while themselves rarely entering the brain, can produce toxins of their own that can affect brain function.

An example is the overgrowth of the yeast organism known as *Candida albicans*, which is becoming increasingly common. This yeast is present in the normal gut, yet if allowed to proliferate it can cause symptoms including bad breath, fatigue, headaches and bloating. A diet that is high in sugar, the saturated fats found in dairy products and red meat, and fermented products such as alcohol, vinegar and blue cheese can encourage *Candida albicans*.

Helping the immune system

A weakened immune system can further encourage the growth of unwanted yeasts, as it is this system that is responsible for dealing with them.

City dwellers are often subject to higher demands on their immune systems, due to the almost constant challenges posed by the number of people with whom they come into contact, as well as the increased pollution and exposure to toxins that city life brings with it.

Nutrient deficiencies can also lead to a compromised immune system. For instance, lack of the vitamin B_6, which is found in abundance in avocados, salmon and brown rice, can inhibit the action of the immune cells that destroy and digest pathogens – the agents that cause disease.

Replacing foods that encourage *Candida albicans* with fresh fruit (although preferably not soft fruit), vegetables (especially dark-green leafy ones, as they contain high amounts of minerals such as magnesium and calcium), wholegrains that are rich in the B group of vitamins, and fresh nuts and seeds (sesame and pumpkin, for example) can support the immune system, allowing it to deal more efficiently not only with yeasts, but with all microbes and bacteria.

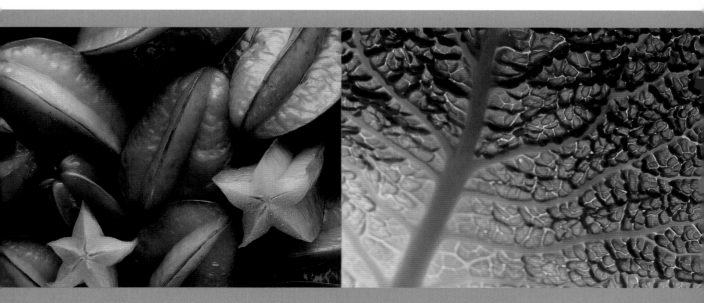

the effects of toxins

Living in the city makes us vulnerable to more toxins than we were ever designed to cope with. Aside from the obvious potential toxins found in traffic fumes, the sheer numbers of people in our cities can lead to increased levels of CFCs (chlorofluorocarbons), which are used extensively in air-conditioning systems, aerosol sprays and household refrigerators. Although the use of CFCs has waned in recent years, the ozone layer above our cities has already been damaged. This is especially true of cities that enjoy warm climates, such as Sydney, Los Angeles and Rio de Janeiro, where air-conditioning is more widely used.

A weakened ozone layer leads to increased levels of ultraviolet light, which in turn increases the incidence of free radicals in the body, which have been widely linked to major diseases such as heart disease and cancer (especially skin cancer).

Meanwhile traffic fumes contain lead. Although lead levels in the air have fallen significantly with the advent of unleaded fuel, lead is still present in the air that we breathe. Lead has been found to block the absorption sites of essential minerals, leading to deficiencies. It has also been linked to behavioural problems, impaired memory and cognitive function. Lead is stored in the bone matrix for up to eight years and can be released at any time.

Aluminium is also found in many seemingly harmless and commonplace products – some toothpastes contain the trace metal, as do some antacids (used to combat indigestion) and water sources.

Allergies and sensitivities

Excess toxins can stress the liver, which in turn can lead to toxins being excreted or stored elsewhere. Toxic overload can also cause increased sensitivity to foods, through a condition known as leaky gut syndrome or increased gut permeability. In this condition the liver is unable to cope with the toxic overload, so toxins are passed into the colon without having been detoxified. This 'dumping' of toxic build-up causes inflammation of the sensitive lining of the gut, leading to increased permeability; this in turn allows partially undigested food particles to

Metal toxicity symptoms

METAL	SYMPTOMS
Mercury	Anaemia, anorexia, depression, fatigue, insomnia, impaired cognitive function, headaches and irritability.
Lead	Anxiety, anaemia, impaired cognitive function, constipation, fatigue and bone pain.
Aluminium	Dementia, muscle pain, gastroenteritis.
Cadmium	Alopecia (hair loss), anaemia, fatigue, emphysema, osteoporosis.

If you have experienced more than three of these symptoms, then you should consider having a hair mineral analysis carried out, which can be arranged for you by a nutritional consultant.

pass into the blood, where they attract the attention of the immune system, causing either an allergic reaction or a less severe response, such as a rash or headaches. In this way today's food can become tomorrow's allergens or sensitivities. Toxic build-up can also mean that the excess toxins are stored in the body's tissues and cells.

Many city dwellers could benefit from a hair mineral analysis. This entails taking a small cutting of hair from the nape of the neck and analysing its mineral content, which reflects recent tissue levels of minerals – both those that should be present and those that can pose a threat to optimum health. It is not at all uncommon to find that someone who lives in a city has excessive mercury, aluminium, cadmium or lead in their hair.

'Chelating' foods

Removing heavy metals from the body can be done by including foods that are known to 'chelate' metal. These foods contain substances that bind to the metal and encourage its elimination. Apples are one such food (see also p. 19), as they contain pectin in the peel, which chelates heavy metals. Supplements that act in the same way, such as potassium and magnesium citrate, in addition to vitamin C, may need to be taken for a period of two to three months to ensure that the heavy metal is diminished in the body.

Every day we are exposed to many potential toxins, but the food that we choose to eat can help reduce the amounts that are absorbed by the body. Eating just one fresh apple a day can help chelate heavy metals, such as lead, from the digestive tract.

There are many other adverse factors that can affect the body. Excess or constant noise is a good example – aircraft flying overhead and the continuous hum of traffic are so common that we rarely notice them after a while. While noise pollution does not require traditional methods of detoxification, it does place an extra burden on the body. By stressing the system it can make it less able to process other toxins.

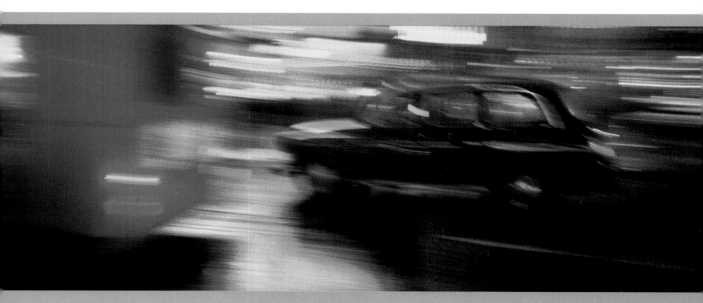

detoxifying:
what happens in the body?

Detoxifying has become a buzz-word and many books have now been written devoted solely to the subject. But do we know exactly what the process of detoxification entails?

As we have seen, the liver is responsible for detoxifying substances after they enter the body. This multi-functional organ is highly evolved, and the detoxification process is but one of many essential roles that the liver performs, including the regulation of blood glucose levels (see p. 50), protein and fat metabolism, and the storage and activation of important vitamins and minerals (the liver stores vitamins A, B_{12}, D, E and K, as well as the minerals iron and copper).

We have also seen (pp. 14–15) that there are two stages in the breakdown of toxins into their constituent parts. The first-stage by-products are free radicals, which can be quashed by vitamins A, C and E, in addition to the minerals selenium and zinc, amongst others.

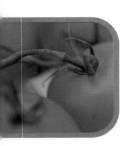

It is vital that we eat fresh fruit and vegetables, nuts, seeds and wholegrains daily, all of which are rich in these antioxidant nutrients. Recent research has also highlighted other antioxidants, such as green tea and a constituent of tomatoes called lycopene. Consumed daily, such foods can support the liver's ability to detoxify more efficiently.

Alcohol and chemicals

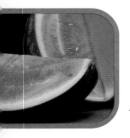

It is important to remember that the liver processes many toxins, including alcohol. Drinking alcohol every day means that the liver has to work harder to handle its workload. If you do drink daily, consider giving your body a break from alcohol (a few weeks if you can, or perhaps a few days every month), or drinking (moderately) only three times a week. This will allow the body more of a chance to free stored toxins and process them efficiently.

Many people who do stop drinking, or reduce their intake, experience minor skin problems and headaches – this is simply a sign that the toxins are being released and processed, and means that healthy liver functions are now taking place. City life inevitably brings with it extra pollution and chemicals, while socializing in a city often involves alcohol intake and/or cigarette smoke (either through smoking yourself or through inhaling cadmium-containing smoke in bars or clubs).

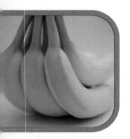

Pesticides that are regularly sprayed on our produce are another hazard; they may be considered within health guidelines to be 'safe', but they still add to the toxic load that requires the liver's action. The same is true of chemicals that are used in processed food. They may be deemed safe because they are used in small amounts, or acceptable because they fall within the allowable range, but our total toxic burden increases if processed or packaged foods are eaten regularly. This is not to say that all processed foods contain harmful chemicals – but many do, and ideally they should constitute only a very small part of our diet, not a major part.

Combating metals

Heavy metals, such as lead and mercury, require the following nutrients for removal:

LEAD CHELATION

Pectin from apples; algin from seaweed and sea vegetables; vitamin C, found in strawberries, citrus fruit, kiwis and potatoes; fibre (found in fruit and vegetables and wholegrains such as oats) can also reduce the initial absorption of lead. Zinc has the same effect, and can be found in egg yolk, fish, oysters, turkey, and sesame/sunflower seeds.

ALUMINIUM

Deficiencies of other minerals allow aluminium to be taken up by the body, so ensure that your diet is rich in foods that contain zinc (see p. 85), iron (found in nuts, some seeds, wholegrain products and blackstrap molasses) and calcium (found in almonds, green leafy vegetables, salmon and soya products).

MERCURY

Mercury is found in some fish and older dental amalgams. Its uptake can be reduced by ensuring that the diet is rich in calcium (see p. 89) and zinc (see p. 85).

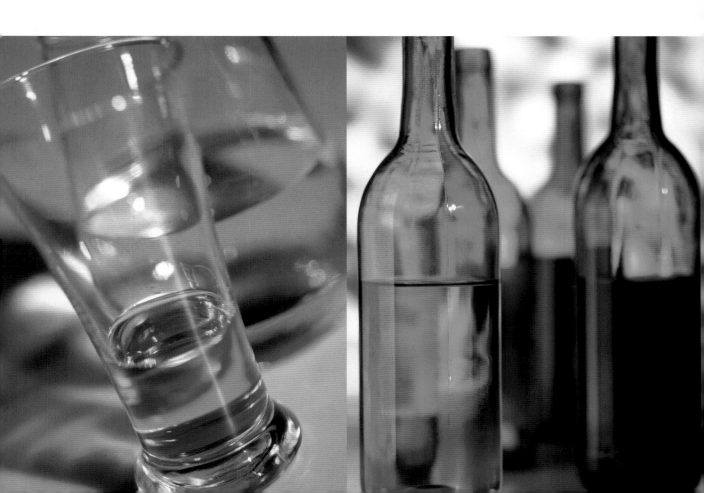

which foods help detoxify
the body

The process of detoxification is a complicated one and is reliant upon many nutrients for optimum function (see also box on p. 39).

Ideally the liver must be supported so that its efficiency is not compromised. It requires a number of specific nutrients for optimum function, including: methionine (from eggs, fish, meat and milk); choline (from cabbage, eggs, chickpeas, lentils, rice, soya beans); silymarin/milk thistle (a herb that can be supplemented under supervision by a nutritional consultant or herbalist); thiols (found in onions, garlic and cruciferous vegetables).

Water

The role of water in the process of detoxifying cannot be overstated. Water is required in every part of the body, not least in the kidneys, which are an elimination route for the excretory derivatives (see p. 16), the end-product of the liver's detoxification process.

At least $1^{3}/_{4}$pt/1l water – and preferably double that amount – should be drunk daily. This does not include fluids such as tea and coffee, which can have a diuretic and therefore dehydrating effect, and can in themselves contain chemicals and pesticides requiring detoxification, further adding to the toxic load. Instead drink still mineral water whenever you can. It is best not drunk directly from the refrigerator but slightly below room temperature, as this is how the uptake of water by the body reaches its optimum level.

Juicing

Juicing vegetables and fruit is a delicious way to ensure that you get the nutrients they contain, in a liquid form that is highly absorbable. However, there is a balance to be struck. Nature gave us the whole fruit for a reason – let's take the example of an orange. This contains, among other things, vitamin C, fructose (fruit sugar), fibre and pith. When eaten whole (after peeling

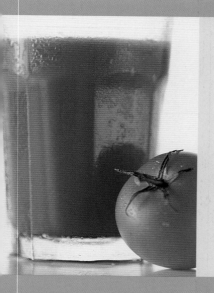

City anti-pollution programme

- Eat plenty of apples for their pectin content.
- Eat seaweed or a sea vegetable at least three times a week.
- Eat zinc- and calcium-rich foods (see p. 85).
- Reduce your alcohol intake or avoid alcohol for most of the week.
- Favour organic products that have not been sprayed with pesticides.
- Eat fresh foods and avoid packaged foods whenever possible.
- Eat plenty of fresh fruit and vegetables that contain vitamins A, C and E, and the minerals zinc and selenium (found in broccoli, bran, mushrooms, wholegrains and garlic).
- Keep your sugar intake to a minimum.

of course), the fibre slows down any blood sugar release, while the pith contains compounds called flavanols, which serve to recycle the vitamin C so that it becomes more potent. All in all, the orange contains all that is required for maximum benefit from eating that fruit.

Once it is squeezed, however, we lose the fibre and some of the flavanols, and some vitamin C breaks down, so while we are benefiting in certain respects, the potential advantages are decreased.

Juicing is a delicious way to ensure that you obtain the nutrients contained in fruit and vegetables in a highly absorbable form, but it is not ideal for everyone.

If you have any problems in balancing blood glucose levels (see p. 50), then juicing may not be for you. For by drinking the juice of fruit and vegetables you are missing an essential element that nature placed in the produce – fibre. Fibre not only slows down glucose release, but also helps in the removal of toxins from the colon. A fibre-poor, yet nutrient-rich diet could have many health repercussions, so it is advisable to consume juice *in addition to* the minimum requirement of five whole portions of fruit and vegetables per day. If you own a juicer, then use it often to make detoxifying juices (see p. 134 for the City Plan juice), but do ensure that you drink these *as well as* eating whole fruit and vegetables.

Raw or cooked foods?

Raw fruit and vegetables contain many substances (not least fibre) that can help in the detoxification process. Cooking – or, more precisely, overcooking – vegetables substantially reduces their nutrient content, particularly that of the water-soluble vitamins, such as the B group and vitamin C. Fibre in vegetables is also broken down by heating. So ensure that your diet contains ample raw foods, such as fresh green vegetables and fruit. For some delicious raw salad recipes see pp. 108–9.

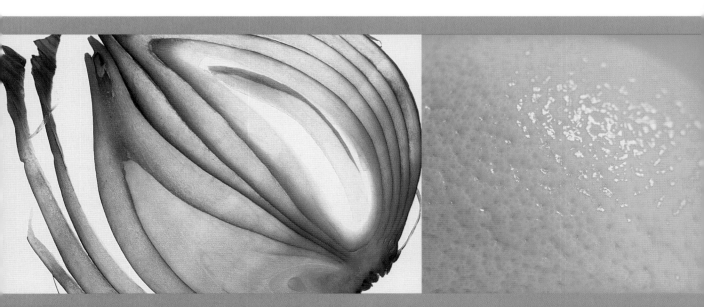

the effects
of the city

We have seen how elements in the food that we eat and the air we breathe need to be detoxified by the body, and how frequent stress can be harmful in the long term. However, many other aspects of daily city life can have a potentially detrimental effect on the body.

City dwellers are likely to spend more time indoors than others – in offices and workplaces – and this carries its own potential health implications.

Office lighting

Indoor lighting has changed considerably over the last few years. Many modern offices now use state-of-the-art lighting, which provides more than adequate illumination. However, some older offices still use fluorescent lighting, or perhaps you work at home and find that your eyes become tired or you develop a headache. This can often be attributed to insufficient broad-spectrum lighting.

Various cells in the eye are sensitive to light. Natural daylight provides the perfect balance so that all types of retinal cells, or cones, are stimulated and receive a balanced picture that combines the three 'shades' of light – yellow, blue and red. The same is true of a colour television, which has settings to alter these colours and, by balancing the three, a natural picture can be achieved.

Artificial light can mimic this colour balance, although many types of lighting provide excessive yellow shades, which overshadow the blue shades. The eye muscle then works to stabilize the imbalance, which can lead to extra strain being placed on the eye and, possibly, to headaches.

Fluorescent light can also cause eye-strain, not least because it does not properly cover the complete colour spectrum, but often emits a higher level of blue light (this explains why fluorescent light seems so 'white'). Furthermore, it sometimes flickers imperceptibly, which causes the eye muscle to almost constantly refocus, leading to continued strain and headaches.

It has also been found that inadequate lighting can lead to an increase in the levels of cortisol (the steroid hormone that is raised at times of stress), due to its natural rhythms being disturbed. Increased cortisol levels have many effects – for the full range of potential health issues relating to this subject see p. 12.

The most effective way to avoid eye-strain and headaches is to change older lighting systems for newer ones that cover the broader spectrum of light (check with manufacturers). Some specialist lighting companies now produce a bulb that flickers at a far higher rate than conventional light bulbs, so that the eye does not strain to refocus. Such bulbs also have an equal range of the three shades of light and more closely approximate to daylight. Obviously such measures may not always be practical, so there are nutritional remedies that can support the eye, both in its function and in its muscle action. Ensure that at least once every two hours you take a few minutes to go outside and let your body and eyes benefit from some natural daylight. This will allow the full spectrum of light into your eyes, enabling them to have a period of respite from artificial illumination. Ensure that you have eyes checked regularly by a qualified optician.

Eye-support

Antioxidants are essential for protecting the eye. The most effective antioxidants are vitamins A, C and E and the minerals selenium and zinc (see p. 39 for antioxidant foods). However, other antioxidant compounds have now been shown to have a particular affinity with the eye – for example, bilberry contains flavanols that protect the sensitive cells of the eye, and which can be either found in the fruit itself or taken in concentrated form as a supplement. Many vitamin C supplements are now formulated with added bilberry extract to enhance their potency.

The herb *Ginkgo biloba* is thought to have oxygen-enhancing properties and, as such, might be included in an eye programme, although it is advisable to seek the advice of a nutritional consultant first.

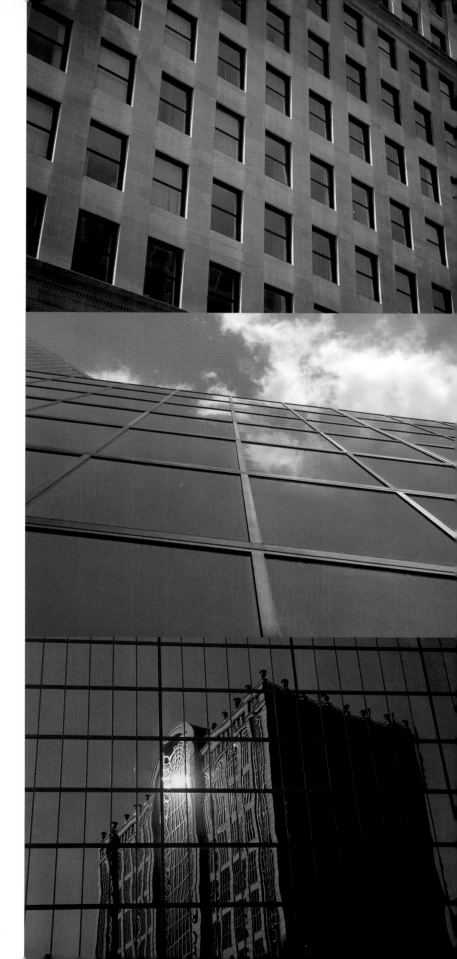

space and sunlight

Space and sunlight are both commodities that are at a premium in the city. Personal space – be it at home or at work – comes at a price that not everyone can afford, so it is important to create some space for yourself whenever possible. For some people, this might mean being aware of how much time we spend indoors, and making time to walk in the park. Perhaps you can combine this with travelling to work (see p. 36). Being in contact with the earth, being aware of the changing seasons and spending time whenever possible in a quiet, relaxed atmosphere can have many benefits.

The immune system benefits from receiving natural sunlight every day – that means direct sunlight, not the sunlight seen through windows or sunglasses. White blood cell production is thought to increase in the presence of direct sunlight, and vitamin D is synthesized by the skin in the presence of natural sunlight. So try to get at least 20 minutes of direct sunlight every day.

Breathing deeply during time spent outside will help re-oxygenate the body – try breathing slowly and deeply, to the bottom of your lungs and holding the breath for ten seconds, then exhaling quickly. Do this three times and note how much more relaxed you feel. An interesting experiment is to take a blood-pressure reading before and after this exercise – your blood pressure is likely to have fallen by as much as ten per cent, which relieves pressure on the heart and the whole cardiovascular system. Most importantly, it can also relieve stress, as it allows the adrenal glands to relax and not have to produce adrenaline. This in turn allows the muscles to relax and glucose stores to remain intact – in short, it will relieve many of the negative aspects of stress.

Indoor environments

Being inside for extended periods of time has other associated health issues. The advent of central heating and air-conditioning systems has resulted in less fresh air circulating in our environment. Oxygen levels are therefore likely to be lower than is ideal, and we are probably breathing in increased levels of carbon monoxide from some domestic heaters and cookers. Tissues with the highest oxygen needs, such as the heart, the brain and muscles used while exercising, are the first to be affected by increased carbon-monoxide levels.

Symptoms may mimic a cold or influenza and may include fatigue, headache, dizziness, nausea and vomiting, cognitive impairment, and tachycardia (rapid beating of the heart). If much of our time is spent inside in a poorly ventilated environment, levels of carbon monoxide could rise leading to hypoxia (a deficiency of oxygen in the body).

However, some indoor health issues are not even as obvious as excess gases. Increased moisture in the air – from cooking, heating, double glazing or refrigerator coils – can lead to microbes and fungi growing under carpets and flooring or on the walls behind kitchen cabinets. Such microbes and fungi are then released into the air that we breathe – and many of them can cause upper-respiratory-tract complications.

Combating airborne organisms

While it may not be practical to clean behind kitchen cabinets, it is possible to ensure that your kitchen is well ventilated at all times.

Nutritionally, it is important to make sure that you do not exacerbate the growth of yeasts and microbes by consuming foods that will encourage them in the body. Once inhaled, these organisms thrive on refined sugars, yeasts and fermented products, including bread, yeast drinks and spreads, vinegars and alcohol (including wine, beer and many spirits), so cut down on these products.

Ensuring that your immune system is fully supported can also assist in combating airborne organisms. Concentrate on foods that include the following nutrients: vitamins A, C and B_6, plus the minerals magnesium, calcium, selenium, zinc, manganese and iron. The majority of these are found in abundance in fresh fruit and particularly in vegetables. Lightly steamed or raw vegetables, eaten daily, can strengthen immune reactions. Add some fresh unroasted seeds, such as sesame or pumpkin, as a snack and you will have the full range of immune-boosting nutrients.

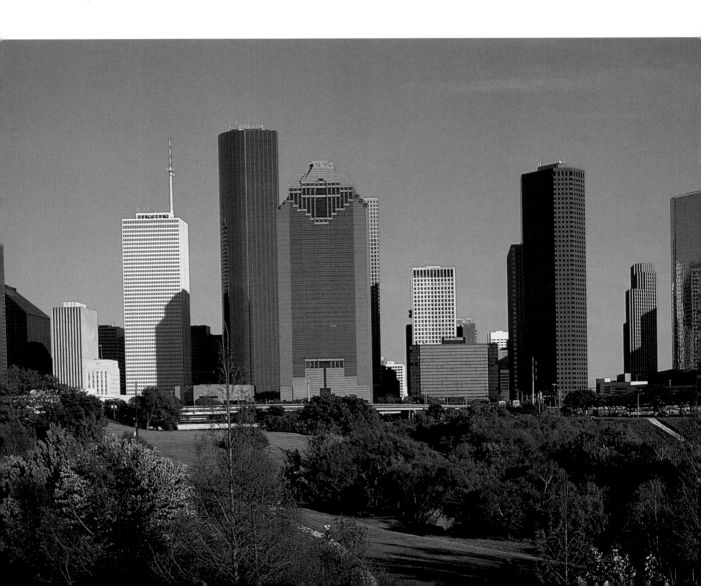

air quality

The quality of the air that we breathe is obviously of great importance. We have already seen how heavy metal toxicity (which includes traffic fumes) can be measured in our body tissues by hair mineral analysis (see p. 17), and again hypoxia is a risk, because carbon monoxide is often found in abundance in both traffic fumes and cigarette smoke.

Most cities have strict guidelines regarding air quality; some, such as Singapore, only allow private cars to enter the downtown area on alternate days, thus reducing by half the potential emissions (however, many people have tried to overcome this by owning two cars that have permits to enter the city on different days!).

Most major cities now publish daily figures showing the level of gases and other elements in the air. For example, figures show that lead levels measured on one of London's busiest roads have fallen by almost 95 per cent since 1983 (linked to the advent of lead-reduced petrol and catalytic converters), and on average carbon monoxide levels have fallen by almost 40 per cent. While this might seem encouraging, increasing car use could in future see this figure climb once more.

Carbon monoxide is a colourless, odourless gas and is a by-product of the normal burning of hydrocarbon fuels, such as petrol. Carbon monoxide emissions are at their highest when engines are first started, or in cold weather, as the production of carbon monoxide is greatest when combustion is incomplete (when starting cars, the ratio of oxygen to fuel is at its lowest, just as it is in cold weather).

Carbon monoxide enters the bloodstream through the gaseous exchange that takes place in the lungs, and combines with oxygen to form carboxyhaemoglobin. This new substance

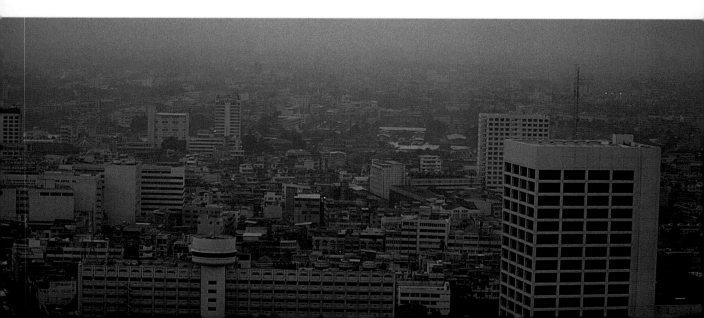

substantially reduces the blood's ability to carry oxygen throughout the body. Excess carbon monoxide has been shown to be associated with fatigue, muscle cramps, nausea and reduction in cognitive function (see p. 24). It is often misdiagnosed as colds, or similar viruses, and treated with antibiotics, which may influence overall immunity.

While modern car engines emit far lower carbon monoxide levels than earlier versions, the presence of the gas in city air may still be considered potentially damaging, for its effects can be cumulative. The best defence we can have is to ensure that we have good levels of antioxidants in our bodies and a generous intake of nutrients from fresh vegetables, unroasted nuts and seeds, fruit and wholegrains.

Cellular/mobile telephones and VDUs

Mobile-phone use increases daily. A few years ago only the wealthy few had access to cellular telephones, but they are now more affordable than ever and have become an essential tool for work and play. As these instruments become smaller and cheaper, more of us are able to enjoy owning our own mobile telephone.

The advent of Internet-compatible mobile telephones will no doubt serve to increase ownership and frequency of use. Furthermore, some countries have progressed to wider-ranging uses for mobile telephones – for example, in Finland users can now order soft drinks and pay for parking meters with their mobiles, with the charges appearing on their monthly phone bill. Such advances will also increase ownership and, with it, the need for more transmitters in every city. These transmitters emit low-level radiation, and while the levels are currently thought to be safe, as new functions are introduced for our mobile telephones it is likely that the number of transmitters will have to rise in order to meet demand.

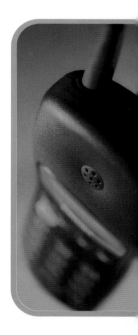

The health risks of having low-level radiation emitted from an antenna held against the head for prolonged and frequent periods every day have yet to be established. The British government recently called for low-level emissions from telephones to be cut to one-fifth of their current level, in line with other European countries, thus highlighting their potential danger. Manufacturers and retailers report that the emissions are well within the limits set by the National Radiological Protection Board, yet research has yet to ascertain how even these accepted power emissions can affect brain cells, when the telephone is held against the head. Until this research has been completed, users would be well advised to exercise caution and not hold the telephone against the head for extended periods of time.

Some experts believe that the incidence of brain tumours and strokes may increase as we use our mobile telephones more often, since many of them are now becoming as cheap as normal land-lines. Some telephones have higher emission levels than others, but even the safest phones involve some radiation emission. How safe is this, and can we protect ourselves in a nutritional way from low-level radiation?

Many children use mobile telephones on a regular basis, yet they have been identified as being at high risk, because their sensitive brain tissue is not fully developed. Does your child include foods in his or her daily diet that can assist in the prevention of tumour growth? Does he or she consume large amounts of sugar and saturated fats, which can inhibit the functioning of the immune system?

What is the best way to reduce the potentially harmful effects of low-level radiation? And is the same true for the radiation emitted by standard VDUs (such as computer screens), which have likewise become an integral part of daily life, in everything from home computers to televisions and computer games?

Reducing radiation

The electrical current that mobile telephones generate is thought to influence blood flow in the brain, which can lead to an increased incidence of strokes. Low-level radiation emissions are thought to pierce the skin and pass through right into the cells, where they can alter DNA (deoxyribonucleic acid, the genetic substance in the cell that is able to replicate itself exactly, so that each new cell has the same DNA sequence). DNA forms the blueprint from which new cells are produced, and damaged DNA leads to damaged cells being produced, which can clump together to form a tumour.

A consumers' report published in Britain claimed that earpieces can act as an added aerial, which in the case of some telephones tested increased radiation emissions by up to 300 per cent. Although this statistic has been refuted by manufacturers, until the facts have been established users should exercise caution when using hands-free mobile phone kits and should keep the telephone antennae well away from the side of the head where possible. There are also some products that claim to absorb much of the radiation emitted by cellular telephones, so consider investing in one to place on the side of your telephone.

The levels at which different telephones emit radiation vary widely, and perhaps the wisest move would be to buy a telephone with the lowest possible emissions. The US standard, known as the Specific Absorption Rate (SAR), was applied to the most popular mobile telephones, and the recorded differences ranged from 2.67 SAR to 0.10. The phone with the highest score emitted 20 times more radiation than the one with the lowest score. Telephones with fixed antennae appear to score highest, and those with retractable antennae that can be raised away from the side of the head had lower scores. The newest and smallest telephones scored well, but on a practical level there can be a problem with poor reception. Ask your supplier for details of the SAR rating of your telephone – if it is over 1.0, be aware that you have a telephone that is at the higher end of the scale and take precautions accordingly.

If you are using a VDU regularly, invest in a screen cover, which will filter many of the potentially negative emissions, since it is made of a type of glass that deflects the rays away from the user and back towards the computer. Try to take a break from your computer at least every hour. In addition, protect yourself by giving your body all that it requires to ensure a healthy and active immune system, and make certain that your oxygen levels are as high as possible by breathing deeply and slowly. The body can be further oxygenated by ensuring that the blood cells that carry oxygen through the body are properly formed, which entails eating adequate quantities of iron (found in nuts, wholegrains, brown bread and lentils). Also invest in an ionizer, which creates positive ions to balance the negative ions produced by electrical equipment.

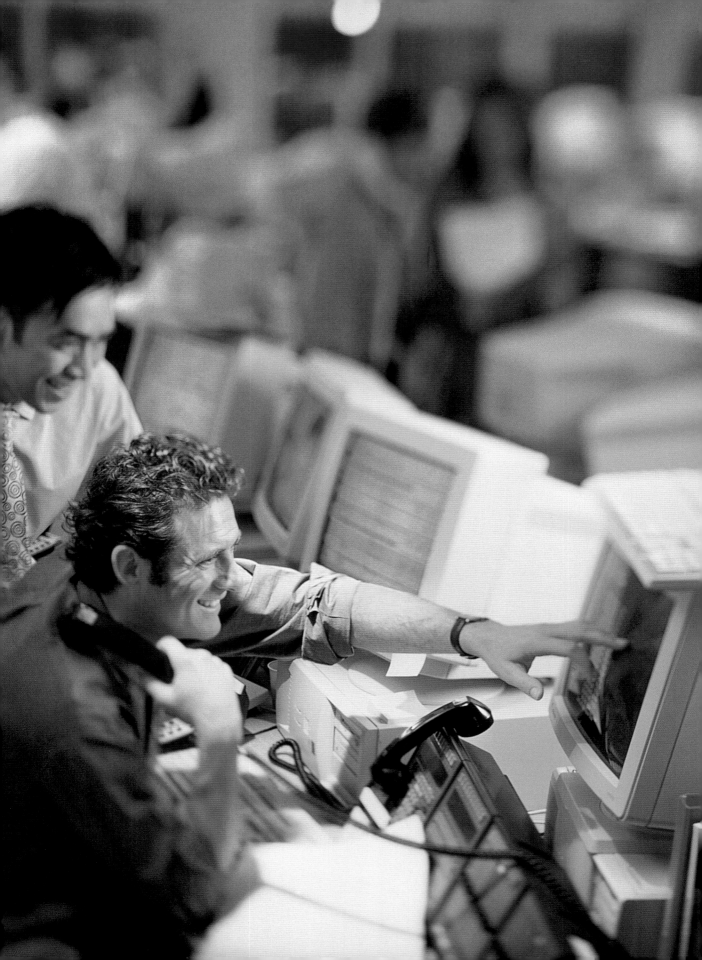

travel foods

When we are on the go all day, relying solely on street cafés and coffee shops for food can interfere with our blood sugar management, digestive capability and immune system, if we do not choose our foods wisely.

Understanding how blood sugar levels fluctuate throughout the day is essential for knowing how best to eat, as it has a direct influence on how we feel. Combining this with immune-boosting and toxin-fighting foods can improve the way we function, both emotionally and biologically. See p. 50 for a full explanation of blood sugar management and how to control this yourself, to your own advantage.

However, there are foods that you can buy from any store or café to improve city life. Let's look at a typical day in the city for someone who is busy and/or working in an office. Having had no time to have breakfast at home, he or she may well call into one of the ubiquitous coffee shops and buy a cappuccino and a muffin or pastry. While this may taste good, the energy that it provides is very short-term and almost guarantees that within an hour or two another coffee and something else sweet will probably be required.

Breakfast boost

The first point is that skipping breakfast is the worst way to start the day. Even having one piece of fruit, such as a banana or an apple, as you dress will help stave off extreme hunger and allow you to make better food choices during the morning ahead, instead of allowing your blood sugar levels to drop, forcing you to choose foods that will offer 'quick fixes'. Eating breakfast is an essential part of the City Plan (see p. 56).

Breakfast on the go

Here are some examples of the best way to enjoy breakfast if you eat while on the run:

COFFEE SHOPS	CAFÉS	TAKE-AWAY STORES
Granola bar	Scrambled eggs	Yoghurt
Fruit	Toast	Fruit shake
Peppermint tea	Tea without milk	Oat bar

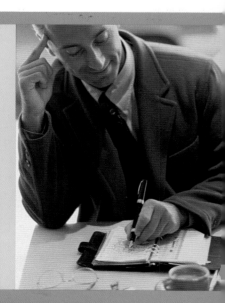

Instead of the coffee and the muffin or pastry (think of what a muffin is: a piece of cake that has been marketed as a breakfast treat – and although cake at breakfast might sound appealing it has no place in improving your health), you could have some peppermint tea, which is also generally available in coffee shops. See the chart on p. 30 for alternatives to muffins or croissants.

Drinking caffeinated drinks all day can deplete vital nutrients such as magnesium and vitamin B₅.

If you feel that you must have coffee in the morning, then limit yourself to one a day, savouring the taste, and do not add sugar. If you have a cappuccino, choose a small one and forgo the chocolate powder on the top: sprinkle some cinnamon or nutmeg on it instead, both of which are sugar-free yet add an interesting flavour to the coffee.

For the journey home, avoid blood sugar lows by having something light to eat before you set off, such as a piece of fruit or a sugar-free flapjack (see p. 37 for snack ideas).

Anti-stress nutrients

Travelling around any city can be stressful, but many foods contain specific nutrients that are required to help the body handle stress. As we saw on p. 10, the adrenal glands respond to stress by releasing adrenaline, which in turn releases stored blood sugar for energy; this triggers the release of the hormone insulin to ensure that blood sugar levels do not rise too far.

So which foods can combat the negative effects of stress? The primary nutrients that are required in higher amounts for city life are magnesium and vitamin C. Both support the adrenal glands and are required in abundance. Coping with the rush hour and using public transport – rushing to catch the bus or train, for instance – are typical of the stresses that city travel can bring with it.

Stress-busting foods

MAGNESIUM-RICH FOODS	VITAMIN C-RICH FOODS	VITAMIN B – RICH FOODS
Almonds	Citrus fruit	Green vegetables
Cod	Strawberries	Brown rice
Soya beans	Potatoes	Dairy products
Sunflower seeds	Berries	Eggs
Nuts	Peppers	Liver
Dark-green leafy vegetables	Blackcurrants	Wheatgerm
Blackstrap molasses	Kiwi fruit	Sunflower seeds
	Cauliflowers	Soya beans
	Guavas	Lentils
	Mangoes	Corn
	Papayas	

foods for the
glove compartment

Many of us use our cars seemingly all day. From school runs, shopping trips, running errands or delivering goods to driving to work or travelling on motorways, the car has for many people become an extension of the home.

Driving around a city can have many hazards, and those of us who do so regularly know all too well how stressful it can be. While the heightened alertness that stress brings with it (adrenaline release is responsible for this – see p. 10) is useful, we can all too easily become irritable and angry. Sitting in traffic also brings with it increased exposure to traffic fumes that can contain lead and carbon monoxide. The foods that we eat during the day should ideally reflect this heightened exposure.

Instead of relying on food stores and cafés, why not think ahead and take some snacks with you? If you are in and out of the car all day, then having any of these beneficial foods in your glove compartment will see you through the day, providing a good alternative to caffeine, carbohydrates and sugar. They also contain many of the nutrients that are required to support the adrenal glands and balance blood glucose levels to keep you awake and alert (see pp. 50–51), as well as protect the body from toxins and assist in detoxification (see p. 18).

Any of the suggested foods for the car, eaten separately or perhaps combined (spread the hazelnut butter on the oat cakes, or have the apple with some seeds or nuts), will make an excellent snack, providing you with some carbohydrates and either some fibre (from the apple) or some protein (from the nuts, seeds or hazelnut butter). Fruit is always a good fall-back, and an apple, pear or banana should stave off hunger, while providing fibre, vitamin C and antioxidant compounds. Your blood sugar is then more likely to stay within the correct range,

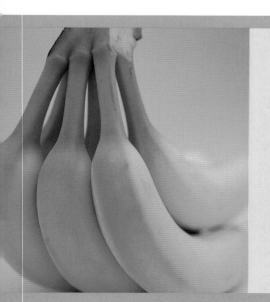

Foods for the car

Here are some foods that combine the beneficial food groups:

Oat cakes

An apple

A bag of unsalted raw almonds

Unsalted raw cashews

A jar of hazelnut butter (without added sugar or salt)

A bag of mixed raw pumpkin, sesame and sunflower seeds

An unsweetened oat flapjack

A banana

avoiding the highs and lows – the roller-coaster syndrome – described on p. 50, and should keep you away from the caffeine and sugar trap.

Road rage

Sadly, road rage has become a familiar part of driving today. Stress levels and tension can run so high that tempers boil over easily, leading to unnecessary aggression. Staying calm is obviously the key to avoiding road rage, and cutting out tea, coffee and sugar will go a long way towards achieving this. Replace them with soothing drinks, such as peppermint and camomile tea, or diluted fruit juice.

Eat little and often to avoid energy lows; make sure, too, that you do not set off on your journey having had only a high-carbohydrate meal, such as toast and cereal. Instead, balance this with a good protein source, such as eggs, and with the fibre found in fresh fruit, oats and wholegrains.

Drinks

It is vital to ensure that you get adequate quantities of water during the day, as it is the primary fluid used to clear toxins from the kidneys. Always keep a bottle of still mineral water in the car. If you find plain water unappealing, add some freshly squeezed lemon or lime juice to it, to give it extra interest (see p. 89 for other suggestions).

While caffeine has its uses, relying on it to stay alert on long journeys is not advisable. First, the energy it provides is short-term and you will almost certainly feel tired within an hour or so. Second, most caffeinated drinks act as a diuretic, so motorway journeys are bound to be interrupted by more stops at service stations.

On long journeys ensure that you stop regularly – every hour, if practical – and walk around a little, breathing deeply and slowly. This can have a more positive effect on mental alertness than a cup of coffee will.

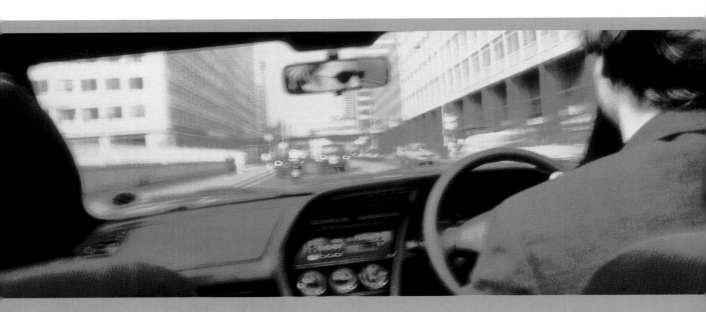

cycling

Cycling is an ideal way to experience the city, and it provides excellent cardiovascular exercise. It also reduces the need for cars, thus lowering pollution and the burden of cars on already clogged city-travel infrastructures.

Increasing numbers of cities are actively encouraging the use of bicycles by providing special cycle lanes. In some forward-thinking Dutch cities, such as Amsterdam, the authorities have instigated a system whereby you can pick up a public bicycle at a designated cycle stop, travel to your destination and leave the bicycle at another cycle stop, ready for the next person to use.

Cycling does have its dangers, however. Apart from being more vulnerable to accidents, cyclists also risk greater exposure to traffic fumes containing lead and carbon monoxide. Many cyclists now wear a protective mask that filters the air – after a day in the city it is alarming how discoloured the fabric that constitutes the filter can become. It would be interesting – and probably revealing – to compare the level of toxic or heavy metals found in the tissues of a cyclist with those of a car driver.

The same principles apply to cycle travel as to car travel, although the need for detoxifying and protective foods is increased. As the action of cycling demands extra oxygen, cyclists are likely to breathe harder to meet the demands of aerobic exercise. Deeper breathing increases the inhalation of traffic fumes, so the role of foods in detoxifying and assisting the liver in its work is especially important.

Aerobic exercise also creates an increase in the incidence of free radicals, as these are a natural by-product of metabolism. As the body's metabolic rate is higher during exercise, this leads to extra demands for antioxidant compounds in order to combat the raised levels of free radicals.

As a cyclist, you could include a few of these foods in your rucksack. Eat an apple before you set off on your journey, and ensure that you have plenty of raw vegetables with your lunch. If you are making lunch at home to take with you, include some protein, fibre and carbohydrates in your lunch box – perhaps some chicken, salad leaves and raw broccoli, peppers and cabbage, some brown rice or a few strands

Ideal cyclist foods

The following foods have been chosen because they contain good levels of antioxidants, are rich in fibre, assist in detoxifying, support the liver and provide balanced energy:

Apples
Pears
Cashew nuts
Almonds
Sunflower seeds
Citrus fruits
Strawberries
Pumpkin seeds
Raw vegetables

of pasta, all mixed together. Using the City Dressing (see p. 122) will further ensure that you get a good supply of the essential fats that are required for efficient metabolism.

If you are buying lunch from a café, try a baked potato with tuna – the potato is rich in carbohydrates for energy, as well as the antioxidant vitamin C, while the tuna provides first-grade protein together with vitamins B_{12} and B_3.

Fluids

Cycling in a city can dehydrate the body, and the extra toxins to which you are potentially exposed further increase the need for water. It is imperative that you take a bottle of water with you – still mineral water is best, but you may want to mix in a little fruit juice for added interest and energy. The juice should constitute no more than 40 per cent of the liquid.

Drinking caffeinated beverages, however tempting they may be, provides very short-term energy and can dehydrate the body. The sugar they often contain can have a negative effect on magnesium, which is an essential component of the stress reaction.

Lite or diet versions of popular drinks can have a similar effect, added to which the chemical used to sweeten the drink requires detoxification by the body, placing an extra burden on the liver, which ideally should be left to cope with the toxins in city air. Likewise, sports drinks are not ideal, for they provide very short-term energy and should be used sparingly.

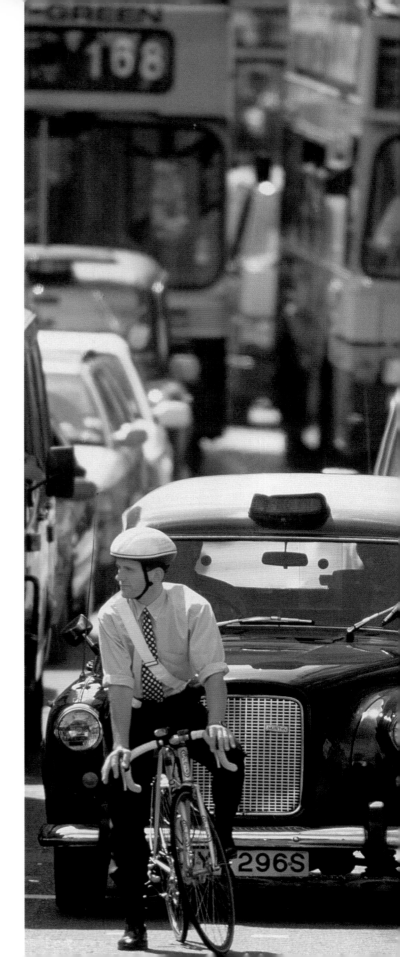

walking

Walking is another perfect way to see a city. Have you noticed that when you are visiting another city you are probably quite happy to walk distances that you would not dream of walking at home in your own city?

Being on foot means that you take different routes, possibly through pleasant parks and squares that no car can enter. Many people express surprise at how beautiful their own city is, when they take the time to walk a little more. Walking also provides gentle exercise and relieves the burden on overcrowded transport systems, but as city dwellers we seem to have less and less time to indulge in walking.

However, walking in any city can bring with it an increased potential exposure to pollution, especially if you walk along busy roads. This in turn requires specific foods in order to help the body detoxify these potentially damaging elements.

Ensure that you have a small bottle of still mineral water with you as you walk, to help the detoxification process and provide adequate hydration at all times. Make certain that you refill it when you reach your destination.

When to eat?

The simple answer to this question is to eat when you feel hungry. Make sure that you read all about balancing your blood sugar levels (see p. 50), as this is a key element in appetite regulation.

If you are about to set off on a journey – be it on foot, by bicycle or in a car – then make sure that you have eaten something shortly beforehand that will keep up your energy levels and alertness for the duration of the journey. Depending on your schedule, this may mean ensuring that you have breakfast every day, or a small snack every two or three hours.

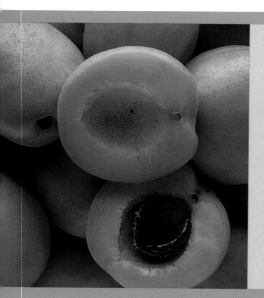

Foods for walkers

Make sure you include the following foods in your daily regime to assist your liver to carry out its function at optimum levels. Many of these foods will also help support your immune system:

Apples	Beetroot
Seaweed	Squash
Pumpkin seeds	Tomatoes (raw)
Spinach	Apricots
Cabbage	Nettle tea

Snacking

It is important to combine carbohydrates, protein and fibre whenever you eat. See p. 52 for an extensive list of meal ideas, but here are some snack ideas that have been designed to keep your blood sugar levels on an even keel:

Rice cakes with tahini

Half an avocado

Frozen apricot and banana shake

Oat cakes spread with hazelnut butter

Fresh fruit salad with live, bio unsweetened yoghurt

Cottage cheese on rye toast

Apple and soya milkshake

Mackerel pâté with toast

Blue corn chips with tomato and chickpea salsa

Boiled eggs with rye bread

You may want to take a small snack with you in your briefcase or rucksack, so that you can eat healthily and appropriately for your particular day. If you do stop in a café, then concentrate on selecting sugar- and caffeine-free items, such as peppermint or spiced apple tea instead of coffee, or plain yoghurt and a piece of fruit instead of a pastry.

Depending on your individual metabolism, your blood sugar levels should then stay within acceptable ranges for two to three hours. The key is to plan ahead. Don't make food choices out of sheer hunger. Instead, try to be kind to your body and your energy levels; follow the principles of the City Plan (see Part 2) and you should experience increased energy and vitality – both of which are essential for successful city living.

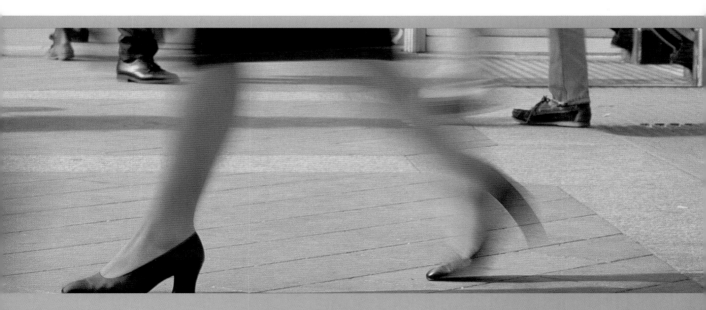

protective foods

Cancer forms from one or more damaged cells that multiply to create a clump of similarly damaged cells. The cancerous tumour then needs to tap directly into the bloodstream for its nutrients, so that it can exist independently of the surrounding tissues.

Some foods and fluids have been found to reduce the likelihood of tumours forming their own blood and nutrient supply: a process known as angioneogenesis. For example, recent studies have identified green tea as having such properties, so including green tea in your daily diet (preferably by replacing tea and coffee with warm or iced green tea) may substantially reduce potential tumour growth.

Many foods are renowned for containing substances that can potentially reduce cancer growth. For example, broccoli is rich in nitrogen components known as indoles, which are known for their anti-cancer properties. The majority of such foods are fruit and vegetables (particularly cruciferous vegetables, such as cauliflowers, radishes, cabbage, turnips and kale) and, while the rule has always been that we should eat at least five portions (or pieces) of fresh fruit and vegetables daily, it might be wise to increase this if you feel that you are at risk of getting cancer. As the incidence of cancer is growing – to the extent that by 2005 half of us can expect to get some form of cancer during our lives – it is more important than ever to include masses of fruit and vegetables in our daily food programme.

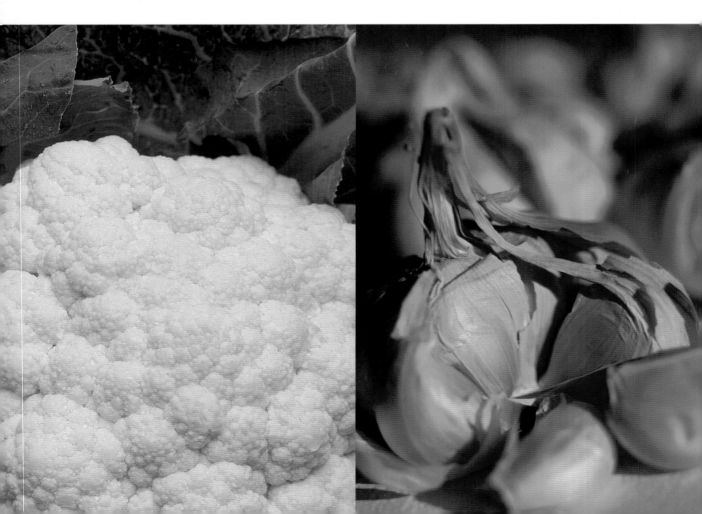

'The future is food'

Dr Richard Gaynor, head of oncology at the Strang Cancer Prevention Center in New York, was recently quoted as saying in relation to cancer prevention, 'We have seen the future, and the future is food.' Scientists have yet to identify all the beneficial substances in fresh produce, but those that we do know about are powerful in promoting health, not least as part of city life.

Recent research has discovered that the darker the fruit or vegetable, the higher its anti-cancer properties are likely to be. For example, research at Glasgow University in Scotland has highlighted the difference between red and white grapes. The red variety offers a far higher level of flavanols than its white counterpart. Its darker skin colour has evolved as a natural way for the fruit to protect itself from the free radical production linked to the sun's rays. Being in direct sunlight has caused the vine to screen itself with a darker skin, and the beneficial properties of these protective measures are available to us as well.

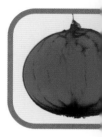

Darker fruits, such as plums, blackberries, blackcurrants and red apples, also offer higher degrees of protection, while vegetables like aubergines, carrots, tomatoes and peppers contain high levels of cancer-fighting nutrients. And some varieties of tomato have been found to contain a higher proportion of lycopene, a potent antioxidant.

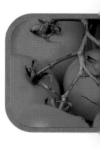

This is not to say that we should only eat darker produce – all fruits and vegetables contain essential vitamins and minerals that should be eaten daily. Add some soya products, such as tofu or soya milk, together with some fresh seeds, such as sesame or pumpkin, and you should provide yourself with a broad range of cancer-fighting substances.

Antioxidant foods that assist in detoxification

As we saw earlier (see p. 20), foods also play an important role in protecting the body by helping in the detoxification process. The following foods have antioxidant properties, contain nutrients that the liver requires or have high levels of fibre:

FRUIT	VEGETABLES	GRAINS	PROTEIN
Apples	Potatoes	Millet	Salmon
Kiwi fruit	Kidney beans	Oats	Egg
Avocados	Chickpeas	Rye	Chicken
Tomatoes	Beetroot	Quinoa	Soya
Bananas	Squash	Sunflower seeds	
Apricots	Asparagus	Buckwheat	
Pears	Sea vegetables	Flaxseed	
Blueberries	Brussels sprouts	Wholewheat	
Figs	Sweet potatoes		
	Carrots		
	Onions		
	Garlic		

troubleshooting

SUBJECT	SYMPTOMS/ PROBLEMS	REMEDY
Toxins	How best to minimize effects	Drink plenty of water; eat fresh fruit and vegetables every day, especially apples and seaweed; include oats in your diet at least three times a week.
Detecting toxins	Skin problems, tiredness, headaches	Undertake a detoxification programme slowly and at a time when you can easily rest, such as a weekend. Mild headaches or a dry mouth are not uncommon side-effects.
Excessive juicing of foods	Hunger, light-headedness	Juicing fruit and vegetables can easily interfere with blood glucose levels, so if you do experience any of these symptoms then juicing may not be for you; for many people, however, it is an excellent way to absorb a high level of nutrients.
Water	Continued thirst	We all need to drink at least $2\frac{1}{2}$–$3\frac{1}{2}$pt/1.5–2l of water daily, but if no amount of water will satisfy your thirst and you find that you urinate frequently, you may have a problem with blood glucose levels, so consult a health professional to test this for you.
Computers	Spending time at...	No real danger has yet been pinpointed, but electrical equipment gives out negative ions, in addition to some low-level radiation. Invest in a screen guard, eat plenty of fresh fruit and vegetables, take an antioxidant compound supplement and perhaps even get an ionizer for the workplace.

SUBJECT	SYMPTOMS/ PROBLEM	REMEDY
Smoky atmospheres	Headaches, breathing problems	Increase your intake of antioxidants in the form of fruit and vegetables, supplements and green tea. Ensure that you get as much fresh air as possible.
Stress	Anxiety, irritability	Eat plenty of foods that contain vitamin C, such as kiwi fruit and strawberries, plus vitamin B_5 foods including sunflower seeds, soya beans and eggs. Magnesium is also important and can be found in green vegetables and fish.
Driving	Lack of time to eat, pollution	Keep some foods in your glove compartment, such as unsalted, unroasted nuts, an apple and a bottle of water.
Walking	Exposure to traffic fumes	Reduce your exposure to pollution by avoiding busy roads where possible, and help your body deal with potentially toxic airborne elements by including plenty of fruit and vegetables in your diet, as well as oats and wholegrains.
Cycling	Aerobic exercise amid traffic	Drink plenty of water, and protect yourself from pollution with a high-fibre diet, preferably from unpeeled fruit and seaweed.

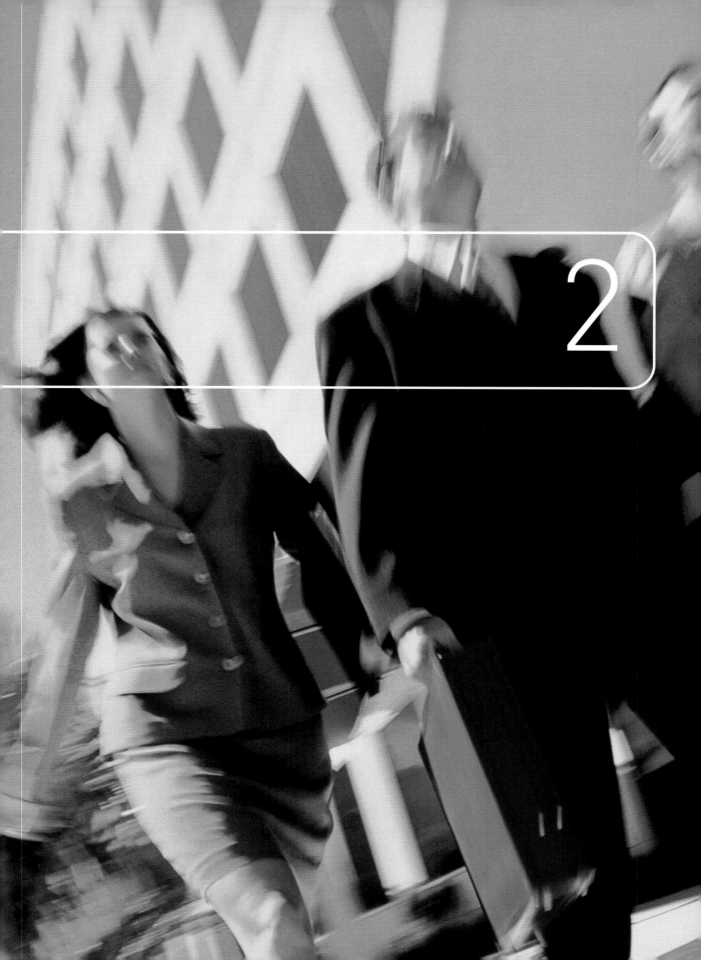

2

the
city plan

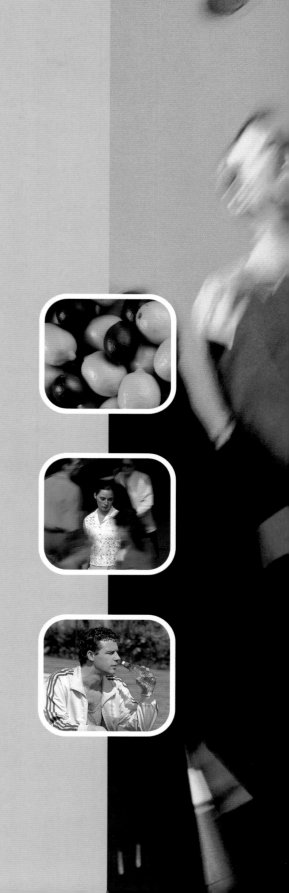

lifestyle questionnaires

The questionnaires that follow have been devised to enable you to highlight areas of your health that nutrition could help to improve.

Energy and vitality

1   Do you find that you have less energy now than you feel you had in the past?
2   Do you ever feel anxious or tense?
3   Do you suffer from self-doubt or depression?
4   Do you feel like sleeping during the day?
5   Do you frequently drink tea or coffee?
6   Have you used antibiotics more than twice during the last twelve months?
7   Do you crave bread, or yeast spreads?
8   Do you eat chocolate or confectionery every day?
9   Do you eat packaged cereal more than three times a week?
10 Do you smoke cigarettes?

Answering yes to four or more of these questions denotes that your lack of energy is likely to be closely associated with your diet.

Pollution

1   Do you often feel snappy or irritable?
2   Do you feel tearful for no apparent reason?
3   Do you live close to a busy road?
4   Do you drive every day?
5   Do you walk in the city every day?
6   Do you cycle in the city?
7   Do you find that your concentration wanders easily?
8   Do you have any amalgam fillings?
9   Do you smoke, or have you smoked cigarettes regularly?
10 Do you experience any unexplained mood swings or depression?

Answering yes to four or more of these questions implies that you have a raised pollution profile and should consider a detoxification programme.

Food groups

1   Do you often eat cereal (including muesli) for breakfast?
2   Do you eat bread every day?
3   Does your daily diet include sandwiches?
4   Do you eat pasta more than three times a week?
5   Do you eat cakes or biscuits regularly?
6   Do you eat pre-prepared foods?
7   Do you eat sweet food or confectionery three or more times a week?
8   Do you eat pizza often?
9   Do you often eat fast food, such as burgers or deep-fried chicken?
10 Do you regularly have a croissant or toast for breakfast?

Answering yes to four or more of these questions indicates that your diet may contain too many carbohydrates.

Sugar management

1   Do you feel sleepy after lunch?
2   Do you often feel thirsty?
3   Do you urinate frequently, perhaps more than other people seem to?
4   Do you find that you have mood swings during the day?
5   Are you frequently tired?
6   Do you crave sweet foods?
7   Do you drink tea or coffee with sugar?
8   Do you drink carbonated canned drinks?
9   Do you crave alcohol?
10 Do you feel anxious or dizzy if you have skipped a meal?

Answering yes to four or more of these questions implies that your blood sugar is not being efficiently managed.

Antioxidant status

1   Do your gums bleed easily when you brush your teeth?

2   Do you have frequent colds or infections?

3   Do you feel that you are showing signs of premature ageing?

4   Do you eat fewer than five pieces of fresh fruit and vegetables every day?

5   Do you bruise easily?

6   Do you smoke cigarettes?

7   Do you drink alcohol frequently?

8   Do you find that minor cuts take a long time to heal?

9   Do you lack sex-drive?

10   Do you have frequent skin break-outs or blemishes?

Answering yes to four or more these questions denotes that you may well be low in antioxidants.

Stress

1   Do you fail to eat fresh fruit and vegetables every day?

2   Do you suffer from insomnia?

3   Have your fat stores increased little by little?

4   Are you frequently irritable or irascible?

5   Do you feel that you have to be right or to win arguments?

6   Do you work especially hard, perhaps harder than others?

7   Do you feel driven to succeed?

8   Do you find it difficult to relax?

9   Do you suffer from frequent colds or infections?

10   Do you eat processed or fast foods regularly?

Answering yes to four or more of these questions implies that you have increased stress levels, which can affect your health.

Modern toxins

1 Do you use a mobile telephone frequently?
2 Do you work in front of a computer every day?
3 Do you work in an air-conditioned environment?
4 Is your car air-conditioned?
5 Do you travel in the city by underground tube?
6 Do you drink alcohol frequently?
7 Do you work in cramped conditions?
8 Do you smoke cigarettes or spend time in smoky atmospheres?
9 Do you spend time in crowded places?
10 Do you get hangovers after drinking alcohol?

Answering yes to four or more of these questions suggests that you are exposed to modern city toxins on a regular basis.

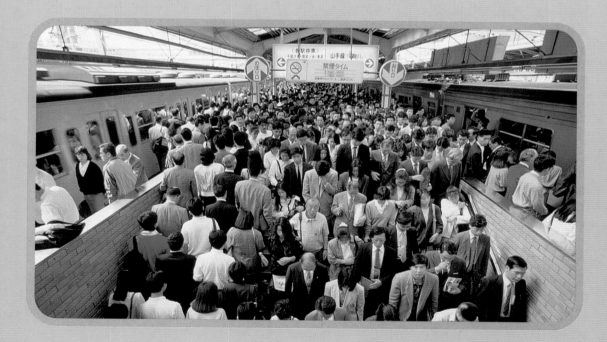

nutrition principles:
why the City Plan works

The City Plan has been devised to combine the best nutritional advice with practical ways to support your body as it endures the special burdens placed upon it by city life. As we saw in Part 1, toxins, pollution, stress and lack of time are all factors that need to be addressed, and the principle of the plan is to strike a good balance between health and lifestyle. This may mean making some changes – for some people this will require only minor adjustments; for others it may involve more effort.

Positive changes in your nutritional status – however small – should benefit your health and enhance your life, for nutrition plays a powerful role in how we feel. When you visit the doctor you are likely to come away with a prescription for a medication that will rapidly deal with your symptoms: all you have to do is swallow the pill. A visit to the acupuncturist, masseur or aromatherapist has even less responsibility attached to it (in addition to pleasure!): all you have to do is lie there while the professional works on you. Nutrition is different: the responsibility lies with you, and you alone, and while the results may be profound, they will be imperceptible at first. After a couple of weeks, however, you should begin to notice the difference.

'Life is for living'

Many people use the 'I could be run over by a bus tomorrow – life is for living' line to rationalize why they ignore their own health. But eating food that has been processed, drinking excess alcohol, smoking cigarettes, eating abundant saturated fats and refined sugar, together with the pollution and stresses that are found in every city, represents the nutritional equivalent of standing in a bus lane wearing a blindfold and covering your ears!

Every area of life is a balancing act (not least what you eat and drink). The City Plan works with you to establish exactly what your personal balance is, while still enabling you to enjoy eating and drinking – possibly with the addition of vitamin or mineral supplements to help you on your way.

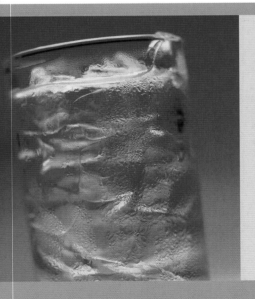

City Plan essentials

The principles of the City Plan are to combine the following nutritional elements:

Blood sugar management
Immune system support
Anti-pollution measures
Detoxifying/liver support
Antioxidant intake
Skin, hair and nail improvement
Vitality and energy
Rehydration
Combating signs of ageing

Most people acknowledge that what we eat is of vital importance, yet do we really incorporate this principle into our everyday lives? Some people still believe that good nutrition is all about lentils and brown rice. This really is not the case – you need to respect your mind and body by providing it with ample nutrients to allow all bodily functions to take place at their optimal level. By replacing the foods that you have come to rely on for short-term 'benefits' with those that can have more profound effects on long-term health, you can easily live without, say, caffeine and sugar.

With good nutrition, many people experience younger-looking and younger-feeling skin, and improved hair and nail quality, not to mention enhanced mental ability and energy. Furthermore, by replacing many of the foods and drinks that have been contributing to health issues with high-quality foodstuffs, you can reduce the potential risk of serious illness, such as cardiovascular disease, some cancers and diabetes.

Many of the health issues that we face every day are exacerbated by city life. The City Plan shows you easy ways to incorporate good nutrition and other lifestyle factors into your daily life in a straight-forward way. It combines the latest research with common sense, taking into account how you choose to live your life, your personal circumstances and simple practicality.

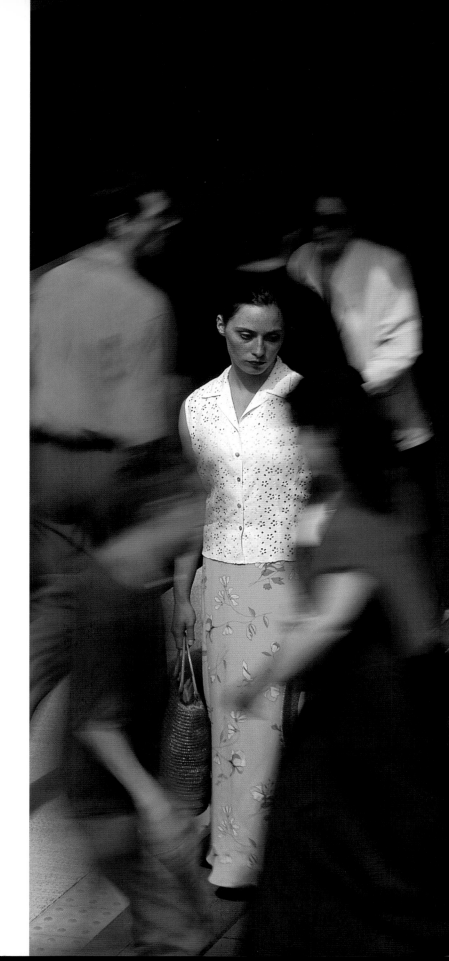

blood sugar management

Perhaps the most important element of nutrition is learning how to control your blood sugar by combining protein, fibre and carbohydrates in a ratio that works for you. Once you have mastered this you will have greater control of your own health than many people believe is possible. The good news is that you can start making changes today, from the very next time you eat or drink something.

Ups and downs: basic metabolism

We all have sugar in the form of glucose in our blood. It is the form of fuel that the body can most easily utilize, and the glucose is derived from the food that we eat. The body has the ability to turn carbohydrates, protein and fat into energy, but the easiest foods to convert are carbohydrates.

Carbohydrates include foods such as pasta, grains, bread, sugar, vegetables and fruit. Some foods (such as refined sugar) are classed as simple carbohydrates, and others (such as wholegrains) as complex, as they are closer to their natural state. Within the carbohydrate group some foods are converted into energy more easily than others. For example, a spoonful of honey releases its energy very quickly, as do alcohol, processed white rice and French bread, which are described as having a high glycaemic value. Oats, basmati rice and raw carrots have a far slower rate of sugar release and have a low glycaemic value.

When sugars are released rapidly from foods they can take your blood sugar to a level at which the body senses there is a potential excess and stores it away, to be used later on. This is done through the action of the hormone insulin, which is essentially a storage hormone. It is released by the pancreas in response to high blood sugar levels in order to bring them down to an acceptable level.

Blood sugar levels influence the way we feel: higher blood sugar can make us feel awake and energetic, while low blood sugar can lead to fatigue, tension, depression and lethargy. However, if blood sugar rises too rapidly we have to produce more insulin, and, if this situation is prolonged, as in chronic stress, the pancreas may become exhausted. Failure of the insulin-producing cells leads to diabetes.

Blood sugar levels fluctuate throughout the day and we all experience them in different ways, but if you can learn to keep your own blood sugar within a tighter band – avoiding the highs and lows – then you are more likely to function consistently. The trick is to make sure that your blood sugar does not rise too quickly, and that it does not fall too sharply or be allowed to stay at low levels for too long. But how is this done?

Controlling your blood sugar

In short, you need to combine complex carbohydrates with fibre and a little protein at every meal or snack. Let's take a typical breakfast. If you eat a bowl of cereal (which is a refined carbohydrate, possibly with sugar already in the recipe), a cup of coffee and a piece of toast, then these are all fast-releasing energy foods, so your blood sugar will climb sharply, triggering the release of insulin, followed some time later by hunger. Many people report that they feel hungry all day if they eat breakfast, and now we can see why.

Had the same breakfast included some fibre, such as an apple (not juice, because this has no fibre in it), a live unsweetened yoghurt (protein) or some scrambled eggs (protein) on toast, then the right balance is more likely to have been achieved. Blood sugar would have risen more slowly, energy would have been more consistent, and cravings for fast-releasing sugars would have been minimized.

Stress and blood sugar

In times of stress, the muscles and liver break down glycogen stores into glucose, releasing it into the tissues to enable the body to deal with the potential danger. Frequent stress – all too common in city life – leads to glycogen being broken down far more often than it was designed to be.

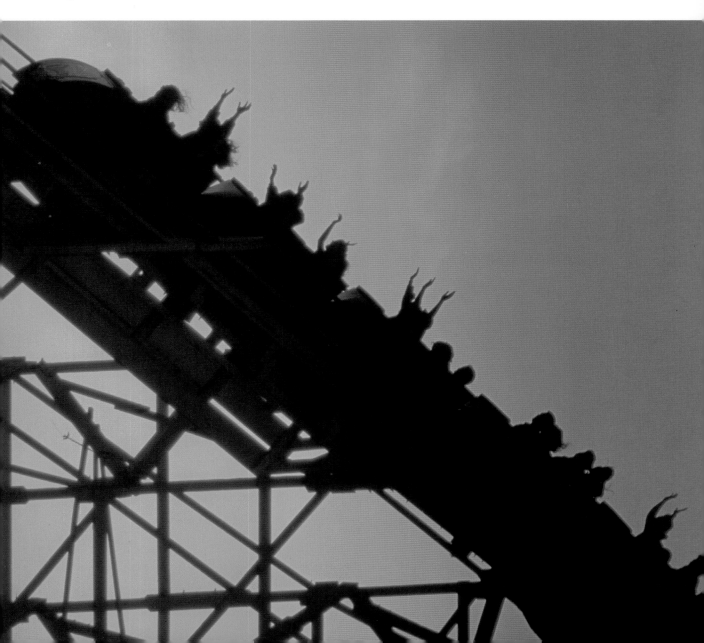

eating at the
right times

Now that we have seen how the food groups interact to affect energy levels, vitality and mood, we will look more closely at what – and when – to eat to maintain your own equilibrium.

Everyone has their own ideal balance of carbohydrates, protein and fibre and the only way to find out what suits you best is through trial and error. Keep a note or diary of what you have been eating and see how that relates to how you feel.

Fibre should be included whenever possible, and because fruit and vegetables contain fibre in addition to carbohydrates they represent the perfect foods. However, the ratio of carbohydrates to protein can influence your blood sugar levels, and it is this that needs to be monitored. Some people feel good on a balance of 1:3 in favour of carbohydrates, while others thrive on greater amounts of protein (such as 1:1). Be careful not to overdo the protein, however, as excessive amounts can lead to an acidic state in the body and increase the risk of osteoporosis.

However, when you eat is almost as important as what you eat. To maintain your blood sugar at optimal levels you will probably need to eat five small meals a day – the rule is 'little and often'.

This might mean that, after breakfast, you should eat a snack at around 11 a.m., assuming that you had breakfast at 7.30 or 8 a.m. With lunch at 1 p.m. and another snack at 4 p.m., that leaves dinner at about 8 p.m. as your fifth meal of the day. You might even consider having a small snack at bedtime.

Ideal snacks

Ideally your snack should consist of something from each column. However, if this is not possible, you could eat something from columns one and two, either together or on its own, but you should never eat anything from column three on its own.

PROTEIN	CARBOHYDRATE AND FIBRE	COMPLEX CARBOHYDRATE
Chicken	All fruits and vegetables contain these	Rye bread
Tahini		Rice cake
Eggs		Oats
Tofu		French bread
Nuts		Rice
Beans		Corn
Yoghurt		Cereals
Cheese		All grains
Soya products		

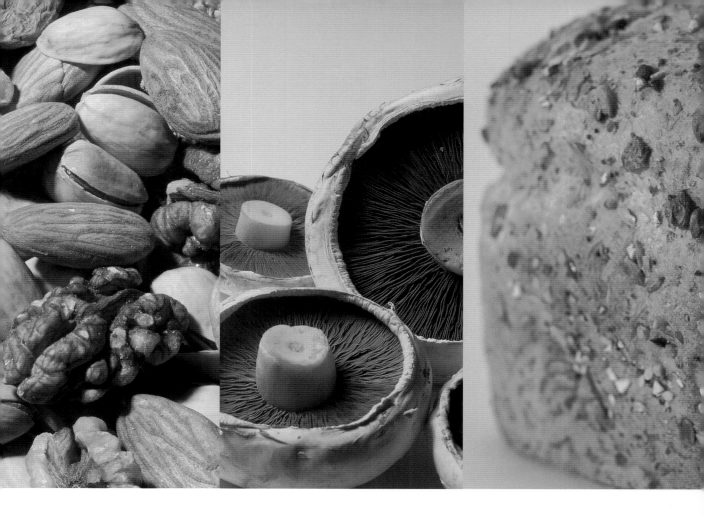

How to snack for better nutrition

For many people, small snacks are better than proper meals! Following the City Plan involves proper snacking; avoiding sugar and caffeine, which provide short-term energy; and including fibre, carbohydrate and protein in every snack, whenever possible.

In addition to energy, snacks should provide antioxidants (see p. 39), chelating substances (see p. 19) and hydration, so the following snack ideas contain all these elements. While a cup of tea or coffee with a biscuit might seem like a good snack at first, it contains no fibre or protein to speak of. Remember that fibre is essential to help clear toxins from the body, so it has added importance in the City Plan.

For example, a rice cake on its own is a rich carbohydrate source, scoring high on the glycaemic index, and could lead to rapid blood sugar elevation. Spreading a little nut butter on it, or some chopped egg, would provide protein, which slows down the sugar release. A bowl of cereal offers only carbohydrates, but by adding in a chopped banana and an apple you get the perfect snack. Better still, the apple contains pectin, which can help remove airborne pollution from the body.

If you choose wisely, and include some fresh fruit or vegetables in your snacking, then you should be able to maintain your blood sugar levels within the optimum range.

a week in the city

What does your typical week consist of? Do you stay home most evenings, or are you out every night? Are your weekends spent clubbing and partying, or do you visit galleries and museums and meet friends for dinner? Do you play a sport, or meet friends to play cards? Do you play in a band or sing in a choir? Do you study or read a lot? Are your weekends an opportunity to exercise and spend time outside, or do you prefer to sleep late and have lazy afternoons in coffee houses? Are you in your twenties and sharing a flat, or living alone or with your family? Do you have children who need to be entertained at weekends?

Just as there is no typical city dweller, so there is no typical city life. Many of us live a combination of all these possibilities. But, however you choose to live your life, nutrition plays an important – if not pivotal – role in enhancing your health.

Forward planning

Whatever you do in your week in the city, try to plan ahead to ensure that you get the best possible nutrition, so that you can carry out your daily tasks with energy and vigour, benefiting from as many of the full range of nutrients as you can. The food choices that you make should be the best ones for you, made from a position where you are not suffering from low blood sugar.

For example, if you are particularly busy one day – perhaps at work or with children – then your blood sugar is likely to be more stable if you eat every two or three hours. However, if you do not eat healthily, or let yourself get too hungry, then any food choices you make are likely to be less than ideal.

When you shop for food, try not to buy just for that day but to think ahead a day or two. When you cook, make some extra for lunch the next day or to add to another meal. This may seem obvious, but many of us find that we have so much to do that we do not manage our time to best advantage. Look at the list of food items that you could buy from a supermarket

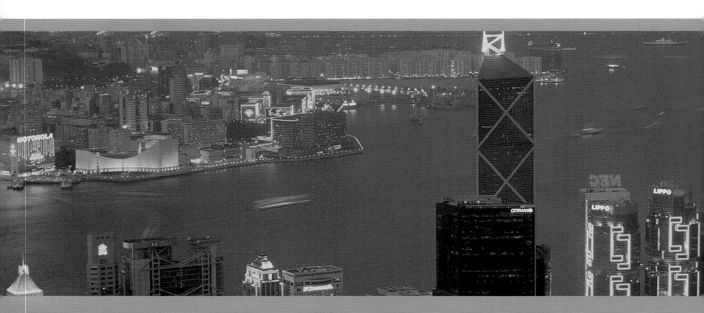

(see p. 62) – perhaps one Sunday when more time is available. These items would combine to provide a number of meals or snacks: either ones that you could prepare in advance or ones that could easily be made at the last minute:

Office foods

If you are at the office, try to keep some foods there that supply good nutrition, together with the right combination of fibre, carbohydrates and protein. You could easily, for instance, keep some fruit in your desk drawer, or a packet of oat or rice cakes and some nut butter or tahini in the office kitchen.

Those of us who work in an office spend a great deal of time there, and what we eat can affect not only our productivity, but also our energy levels and how we feel. Instead of relying on caffeine for energy boosts, learn how to combine foods that will keep your glucose levels more even.

It is not just blood sugar balancing that can help you maintain concentration and enthusiasm at work. The B group of vitamins is especially important in brain function, so ensure that you eat plenty of dark-green leafy vegetables, wholegrains and fish to help boost your mental energy levels. The B vitamins are also closely linked to the health of the gut, in which both beneficial and unfriendly bacteria live side by side. It is all too easy to create an internal environment that can favour the proliferation of the 'bad' bacteria, because they thrive on saturated fats, refined sugars and yeasts.

If your diet contains excess red meat, dairy foods, sugars (remember the hidden ones, too) or bread, then think again. Replace these with fresh fruit, vegetables, fish, poultry, wholegrains and live, unsweetened yoghurt to redress the balance in your favour.

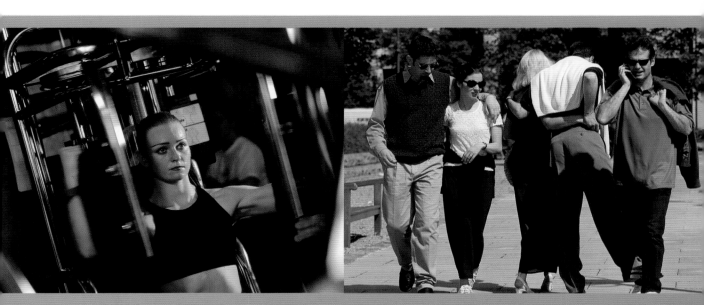

breakfast ideas

We have already looked at some ideas for breakfast (see p. 30) and, having now read all about
the importance of balancing blood glucose levels, you will be able to see why the following
breakfast ideas can work for you. Such combinations embrace the essential nutrients that life
in the city can demand in increased amounts, such as the vital antioxidants that work to quash
excessive free radicals.

Perfect breakfast combinations

Chopped apple with live, bio unsweetened yoghurt and ground sesame seeds sprinkled on top

Scrambled eggs with rye toast

Two boiled eggs with rice cakes or oat cakes and a piece of fruit

Classic City Smoothie (see p. 124)

Rice milkshake with blackstrap molasses and apricots

Millet flakes with yoghurt and apple sauce

Oat or millet porridge with organic soya milk and fresh chopped fruit

Toasted bagel with cottage cheese

All these breakfasts combine carbohydrates, fibre and a small amount of protein. If you do not
have time to prepare any of these, then two pieces of fresh fruit eaten on their own are always
a good standby (a banana and an apple are perfect examples), although you are likely to feel
hungry quite soon afterwards.

Breakfast bars have been widely marketed recently as a good alternative to eating at home.
While they do have some nutritional value, they are very heavy on the carbohydrates and many
contain excessive levels of sugar. There is no good substitute for eating something at home.
Cooked breakfasts are actually not as bad as we might think! If the eggs are scrambled or
poached, and the bacon grilled with the fat removed (or turkey strips chosen instead), then this
contains an excellent balance between carbohydrates and protein. However, cooked breakfasts

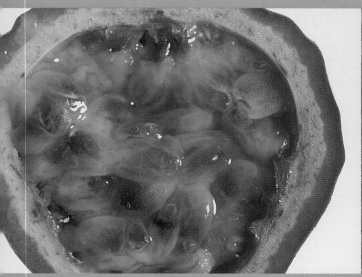
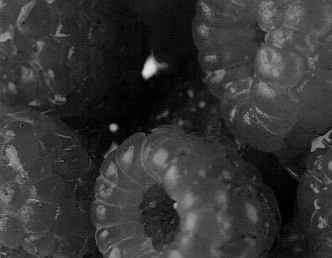

tend to be loaded with fat, so keep them as a treat for the weekend. If you have pancakes or waffles, then forgo the butter and maple syrup, as these are too high in saturated fats and sugar. Instead, eat them with extra fruit (berries, for example) to add interesting flavours.

Breakfast drinks

It is traditional to have tea or coffee with breakfast – indeed, many people feel that they cannot start the day without their favourite beverage. However, the caffeine in regular tea and coffee forces the adrenal glands to produce adrenaline, which in turn raises blood sugar levels and triggers the release of insulin. So both drinks contribute to the 'highs' and inevitable subsequent 'lows', which in turn create the need for more tea or coffee.

While it is true that caffeine can serve to heighten awareness and increase output or performance, that is only true if it is consumed from time to time, and not daily. Many athletes use caffeine precisely for this reason, but were they to drink it all day the effects would be minimized.

Removing caffeine from your breakfast can help you to feel more balanced and focused for longer. Replace it with either green or herbal tea (see p. 88), ensuring that herbal tea is actually made from the leaves of the fruit and is therefore caffeine-free. Many so-called fruit teas are simply regular 'black' tea with added fruit essence; it is true that tea contains flavanols, which are an antioxidant substance (and many teas are now being marketed citing this potential benefit), but fruit and vegetables also contain these compounds, often in far higher amounts, in addition to fibre and minerals.

If you feel you have to have coffee, then have the one cup – savour it, then switch to herbal teas and water (or hot water with a slice of lemon or fresh peeled ginger) for the rest of the day. By the way, decaffeinated coffee does indeed contain very little caffeine, but the chemicals used in the process of removing the caffeine require detoxification by the liver (see p. 86). Try to source a decaffeinated coffee that has been made using the water (rather than solvent) caffeine-removal method, which is usually chemical-free.

Removing caffeine completely from your diet would be ideal, but, as with everything, there is a realistic balance to be struck.

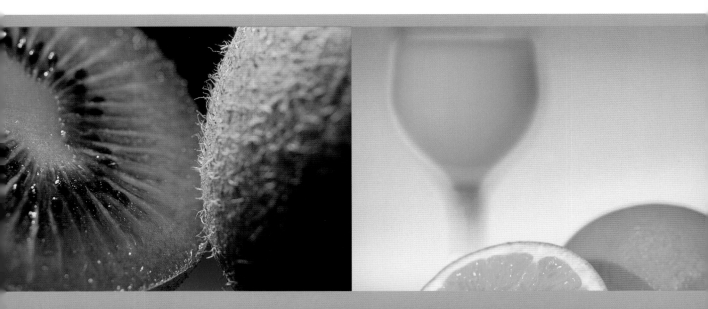

what to eat
to stay alert

It is during the day when we are busy, stressed, or sitting in a meeting or in traffic that our energy levels are challenged. Sometimes you may be in a position where you cannot eat, in which case you should plan ahead (see p. 62 for further information).

Mid-morning snacks

Depending on where you are (at home, in the office, shopping) and how you have spent your morning, you are quite likely to feel hungry by mid-morning. Feeling hungry is a sign that your body is suffering from low levels of blood glucose, and it should be acted upon. In this way the body maintains its equilibrium and you are far more likely to remain alert and energetic.

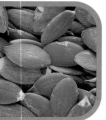

What is the best way to snack, while still maintaining even blood glucose levels? Obviously avoiding refined sugar and caffeine is essential, so the cup of coffee and biscuit or pastry are out. The 'boost' they provide is short-term, leaving you feeling good for a short amount of time, but almost guaranteeing a need for something sweet before lunch. Replace them with foods that provide slow-release sugars, together with a little protein and some fibre. This will keep you going for longer, so that by lunchtime you are not too hungry and can make sensible food decisions, from a position of choice, not cravings.

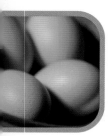

Snacks for home or office

Here are some examples of mid-morning snacks. If you have already had something similar for breakfast, do not choose the same thing for your snack; instead, go for variety. Some snacks are best suited for those at home, but if you are at work you could always make something beforehand and take it in with you. When it comes to the smoothies, why not invest in a blender for the office, dividing the cost between a few of you?

Pear and berry smoothie made with soya milk
Egg and cumin seed spread on rye crackers
Apple and banana fruit salad with unsweetened yoghurt
Pumpkin and sesame seeds with a piece of fruit
Raw cashew nuts and fruit salad
Tofu and apricot smoothie
Oat flapjack (sugar-free) made with fresh nuts
Peppered mackerel on toasted brown or rye bread

Following the guidelines given on p. 52, why not create a few mid-morning snacks that you enjoy, alternating them as often as possible so that you do not have the same thing every day. Ensure that you take the opportunity to have one, if not two, pieces of fruit during the morning, as this is essential in providing antioxidants, fibre, vitamins and many other substances that have yet to be isolated by researchers.

Eating well mid-morning can affect the way you feel for the rest of the day, your productivity and your lunchtime food choices.

Memory foods

Some foods are reputed to enhance memory function, which could obviously be of benefit in the workplace. The nutrient that is thought to be most effective is choline, which is a member of the B group of vitamins and is required in the brain to form the neurotransmitter acetyl choline. Foods rich in choline include eggs, cabbage and caviar. However, nearly all the B vitamins play a role in brain chemistry and can enhance cognitive function, so including fish, chicken, oatmeal and wholegrains in your diet may help you perform better at work.

Top ten tips for office work

Keep your blood sugar balanced.

Get a few minutes of fresh air every couple of hours.

Eat foods rich in B vitamins to support memory function.

Avoid caffeinated drinks, replacing them with diluted juices, mineral water and herbal teas.

Eat lunch earlier rather than later, to avoid poor food choices and cravings.

Bring lunch with you from home if possible.

Do not have the same thing for lunch every day – have variety as often as you can.

Invest in a screen cover to reduce low-level radiation from your computer screen.

Keep a bag of fresh raw, unsalted nuts in your drawer for emergencies.

Eat at least three pieces of fruit during the working day.

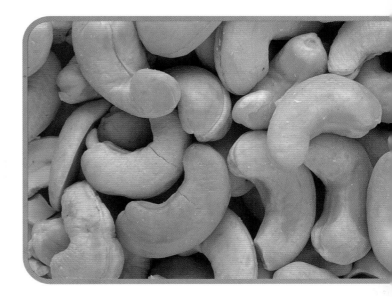

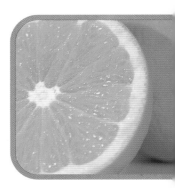

sample scenarios

The City Plan has been devised to work for as many different lifestyles as possible. Below are some sample scenarios with which you may identify.

1. Working from home
Increasing numbers of people work from home, and because of e-mail and the Internet this has become more practical than ever.

Working from home has many temptations and requires a high degree of discipline. Do you find that you wander into the kitchen all too often? Boiling the kettle and picking at something from the fridge may become a way of taking a break and boosting flagging energy levels.

Instead of reaching for the teapot, why not ensure that you have a bottle of water on your desk and sip this throughout the day. You might want to add some lemon or lime juice to enhance its flavour. Switch to herbal teas rather than coffee, and avoid sugared snacks. Ensure that the fridge is filled with fresh fruit and vegetables. Better still, keep some home-made soup there – excellent as a mid-morning snack, or as a larger bowlful with your lunch.

Try the mid-morning snacks suggested on p. 58 – they work just as well as afternoon snacks, especially the smoothies, which supply fructose (natural fruit sugar) to satisfy any cravings you may experience in the afternoon.

2. Housewives/-husbands
The role of the homemaker has often been underestimated. Housework can be tedious, as can the school run. Mothers with young children, or children of different ages, will be all too familiar with the early-morning dash to school, followed by shopping, the gym or meeting friends in the morning, then collecting children from different schools at varying times. Energy levels are likely to flag and keeping up with the demands made upon you is essential. Read all about snacks on p. 58, anti-stress lunches on p. 66 and about driving and 'foods for the glove compartment' on p. 32.

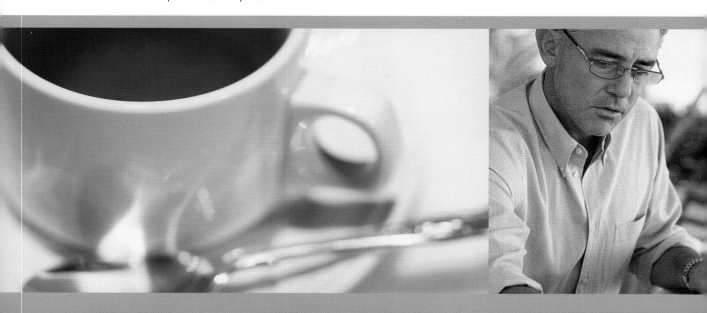

Many mothers say they find themselves picking from the children's plates, or finishing off what they leave, leading to both weight gain and cravings. If this sounds familiar, then it is doubly important that you include carbohydrates, protein and fibre at every meal.

3. Elderly and retired people

After retirement nutrition becomes especially important, as a life spent in the city may have increased the level to which you have been exposed to toxins and free radicals. Perhaps you were in a stressful career, brought up children in the city and have experienced some of the ailments that we seem to accept as inevitable, such as arthritis and fatigue. If so, take advantage of the extra time you now have to shop frequently for fresh produce and ensure that your diet consists of a high proportion of fruit and vegetables. Be adventurous with your food, and avoid falling into the trap of consuming excess sugars and caffeine. Read about balancing your blood sugar (see p. 50) and about free radicals and how to counter them with antioxidants (see p. 39).

4. Working people

Getting up to go to work in the rush hour can mean that breakfast is skipped, or that a carbohydrate-rich breakfast such as toast, coffee and cereal is chosen. This is a sure-fire way to lead to the need for tea or coffee by the time you reach work. While frequent caffeine intake may seem innocuous and traditional, it can interrupt mineral absorption, blood glucose balances and reduce vitamin B absorption, which is vital for energy production at a cellular level.

Once there, you may feel busy and stressed, which leads to the release of adrenaline and in turn to the release of stored blood sugar from the muscles and liver. Raised blood sugar levels then affect your appetite, so that you do not even feel hungry. Have you ever worked on a project with no time to eat or drink anything, only to find that when it is finished you suddenly realize how hungry you are? The stress has kept you going, but when the project is over the adrenaline stops being released, your blood sugar drops and you find yourself in dire need of something to replenish the lost fuel. Eating when you are stressed, even if you just take a few minutes to have some peppermint tea and an apple, or a few almonds and cashew nuts while sitting at your desk, can supply you with a little fuel to keep your blood sugar from crashing after the work is done.

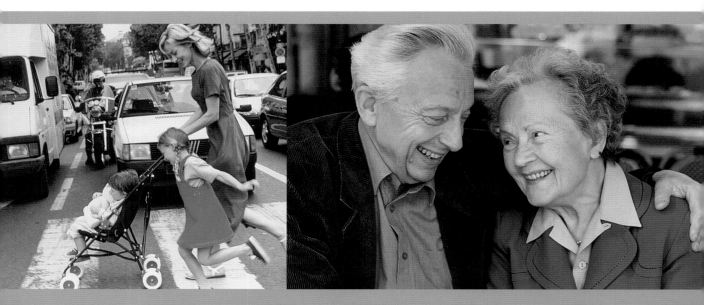

planning ahead

Rather than let yourself get hungry and make decisions about what you are going to eat from a position of low-blood sugar or cravings – or find that your good intentions to eat well have been scuppered because there is nothing in the house to eat – why not plan ahead a little?

What to buy on Sunday

Stock up on Sunday on longer-lasting fruits and vegetables from supermarkets – don't wait until Monday evening, when you're feeling less energetic. Here is a list of just 14 foods that you could easily buy on a Sunday from the supermarket and which could be used in a number of combinations to provide nutrients, carbohydrates, protein and fibre:

Avocados – two	Carrots – six
Eggs – six	Salad vegetables and leaves – a selection
Tomatoes – four	Live unsweetened yoghurt – three cartons
Apples – six	Broccoli – three heads
Rye bread – one loaf	Chicken breasts – four
Oatflakes – one carton	Brown rice – one packet
Pumpkin and sesame seeds – 7oz/200g	Potatoes – two

From this simple list of ingredients you can create:

Quick breakfasts

Scrambled eggs on rye toast

Apple and yoghurt with sesame seeds

Oatflake and apple porridge

Light lunches

Chicken and avocado sandwiches

Salad with raw carrots, broccoli and chicken

Tomato omelette with salad

Suppers

Chicken and broccoli bake

Stir-fry chicken and vegetables

Baked potato with grilled chicken breasts and fresh tomatoes

If you don't like chicken, buy some fish, such as tuna, salmon or cod, favouring fresh fish whenever practical. It is amazing how little we need to change what we eat in order to maximize our health. Even sardines on toast provides fibre, protein, essential fats and carbohydrates!

Remember to snack on apples, pears or any fruit of your choice, plus a palmful of pumpkin and sesame seeds every day.

how to lunch

Many people have to (or choose to!) eat lunch in restaurants during the week. For some people this can be an enjoyable way to meet and entertain business contacts, while others see it as a chore that has to be done. Whatever you think of business lunches, eating out frequently can tempt you to eat too much, or to drink alcohol every day.

Business lunches

Once again, the principles of managing your blood sugar are essential if you have business lunches. A busy morning followed by a dash to the restaurant can mean that you have spent the day so far running on adrenaline. When you arrive at the restaurant your blood sugar, which has previously been kept artificially raised by adrenaline, declines sharply and, as you peruse the menu, you are likely to be making choices from a position of hunger and cravings. In this scenario it is especially important to have had a balanced breakfast (see p. 56 for some ideal breakfast ideas) and a mid-morning snack (see p. 58) to provide you with carbohydrates, protein and fibre. If you have been successful in keeping your blood glucose levels constant, then you are more likely to make positive lunch choices.

Choosing wisely

Let's say that you are in an Italian restaurant. The two columns relating to the Italian business lunch (see left/right) compare typical Italian dishes, but the 'good choices' offer the benefits of antioxidants and blood sugar-managing nutrients, in addition to helping the body cope with the stresses and toxins that you are likely to have experienced that morning.

Italian lunch	
POOR CHOICES	**GOOD CHOICES**
Fried calamari with garlic mayonnaise Roasted vegetables Tagliatelle with ham, peas and cream sauce Wild mushroom risotto	Tomato and mozzarella with fresh basil and olive oil Fennel and avocado salad Grilled salmon with new potatoes and courgettes Grilled chicken with rosemary and vegetables

The 'poor choices' might well be delicious and contain beneficial nutrients, but they can be improved upon. Take the example of the risotto, which is thought of as being a healthy dish. No argument there – the rice contains B vitamins, while the mushrooms contain zinc, calcium, magnesium and vitamins B_3 and B_5. But risotto rice is a white rice and, as such, contains fewer nutrients than brown rice, and as the mushrooms have been well cooked they have little fibre left in them. This dish comprises almost pure carbohydrates, and your blood sugar levels are likely to be disturbed throughout the afternoon, leaving you hungry for sugar or caffeine.

You might even head for the dessert trolley, as you may be craving something sweet.

Had you opted for the grilled chicken or salmon instead, you would have had a first-rate protein source, fibre, minerals and antioxidants from the vegetables (you could even order an extra side-dish of vegetables to ensure that your full nutrient requirement was being met). A few strands of pasta or even some potatoes (not French fries, though) would have given you a carbohydrate source.

The roasted or grilled vegetables that are standard fare in many restaurants will probably have a diminished nutrient and fibre content, due to the extreme heat of the cooking process. If the vegetables are charred, which enhances their look (and some would say their flavour), then they can be potentially carcinogenic, as burnt food can encourage cell alteration in the tissue with which it comes into contact. In addition, the oil in which the vegetables have been roasted or grilled has been heated, thereby making it a potential source of free radicals, so this dish is not as healthy as it sounds.

Of course, life is a balance and food is there to be enjoyed and celebrated, but be aware of the potential health risks and eat accordingly.

Drinking alcohol at lunchtime

Wine (especially red wine) contains antioxidants, and enjoying a glass of red wine with a meal can enhance both the food and the occasion. But drinking wine at lunchtime is almost sure to slow you down in the afternoon, as it has a high glycaemic value, so your blood sugar levels are likely to dip sharply, leading to the need for tea or coffee at around 4 p.m. Furthermore, the sugars in wine can diminish magnesium levels, and as we saw on p. 31, magnesium is an essential mineral in the stress response. And frequent alcohol consumption can diminish the ability of your adrenal glands to cope with stress.

If you do have to eat out as part of your business day, limiting your wine intake to perhaps one glass twice a week can help you function better in the afternoon, as well as improving your stress response.

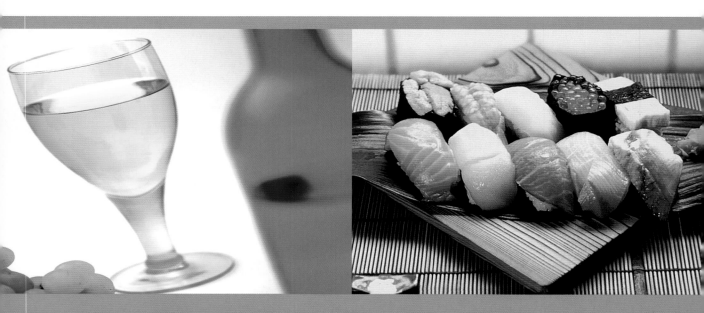

Ideal business lunches

Whether it is Italian food, modern Californian cooking or French cuisine that you have chosen, it is possible to eat out and make good food choices in order to maximize your energy and vitality, without exacerbating stress or fatigue. An ideal business lunch comprises at least two vegetables, either with the main course or with your starter – perhaps a salad with vegetables and some goat's cheese and pine nuts, followed by grilled chicken with a large portion of vegetables.

If you have chosen to eat Thai or Chinese food, then ensure that you do not eat too much rice or noodles without balancing them with some stir-fried chicken, fish or tofu. In addition, always order vegetables, which are usually served crisp in Asian restaurants, thus retaining a high degree of their original nutrient content.

Eating Japanese food is an excellent way to lunch. Sushi combines carbohydrates and protein, with the essential fatty acids in the fish still intact. One drawback, however, is that the rice is white and may contain sugar, in addition to possibly being deficient in some nutrients that are found in greater quantities in brown rice. Japanese vegetable dishes are light and easily digestible, so ensure that you include some of these when you order.

Deli lunches and lunching at home

If you buy your lunch from a deli, as opposed to a sandwich shop or café, then your choice is usually far greater. You could choose to fill a plate or box with different vegetable-based salads, together with some interesting bread. Try a potato salad, with a chicken or fish dish to add some protein, thereby keeping the blood sugar balanced. You might want to buy a little extra, keeping it for an afternoon snack.

If you are eating at home and want a quick, yet filling and balanced lunch, you have the advantage of having a proper kitchen to work in. Soups make excellent snacks, so keep some fresh soup in the freezer and take it out in the morning. Do not have just soup, however, as it invariably comprises only vegetables, with no protein. But you could add some chicken pieces to supply the protein and some noodles for complex carbohydrates.

If you have access to a kitchen at lunchtime, then take this opportunity to prepare fresh foods that are rich in nutrients as these will help you to work well throughout the afternoon.

It does not take long to prepare a salad with some green leaves and some raw vegetables. Shredding or grating raw vegetables makes three or four pieces of, say, broccoli, carrots, courgettes and peppers go a long way. For example, grated raw turnip or sweet potato is delicious and rich in calcium, magnesium, potassium and folic acid, as well as being a good source of fibre. You might want to include a little cold pasta or brown rice to increase the complex carbohydrates. Adding fish, chicken, tofu or even cheese (cottage cheese preferably, as it is low in saturated fats) will balance the carbohydrates with protein. If you do not want a salad, then a simple meal of scrambled or poached eggs – or even sardines – on rye toast will supply a good balanced meal in itself.

anti-stress lunches

Stress is an unavoidable part of life, especially in a city. The potential stresses that we face have increased as technology provides us with new ways to communicate and stay in touch.

When we are stressed, changes take place in the body, as adrenaline is released from the adrenal glands (see p. 10). Specific nutrients, such as the antioxidant nutrients (vitamins A, C and E, plus the minerals selenium and zinc), in addition to magnesium and vitamin B_5, can help the body to cope with stress or reduce the potential hazards of long-term stress.

Below are some food ideas that could help you handle the stress that you encounter. They are all packed with antioxidants and minerals and have been designed to help you keep your blood glucose levels in check.

Signs of stress

When might you need to have a lunch that supplies you with extra stress-related nutrients? During the working week the likelihood of being stressed is obviously increased, but how aware of your own stress levels are you? You may feel calm and capable, but internal stress is a silent problem, one that can manifest itself in any number of ways.

For example, lack of vitamin C will affect your adrenal response to stress. But how do you know if you have a shortage of vitamin C? Telltale signs are a general lack of energy, frequent colds and infections, gums that bleed when you brush your teeth and nosebleeds. You may have one or more of these symptoms because you are stressed, in which case your adrenal glands are rapidly utilizing your vitamin C, which increases your requirement.

A typical lunch for someone who works might be a shop-bought sandwich, a packet of crisps, a carbonated drink and something sweet, such as a chocolate bar or dessert. Hopefully the sandwich will be on brown bread and will contain some protein, such as tuna or chicken, but it

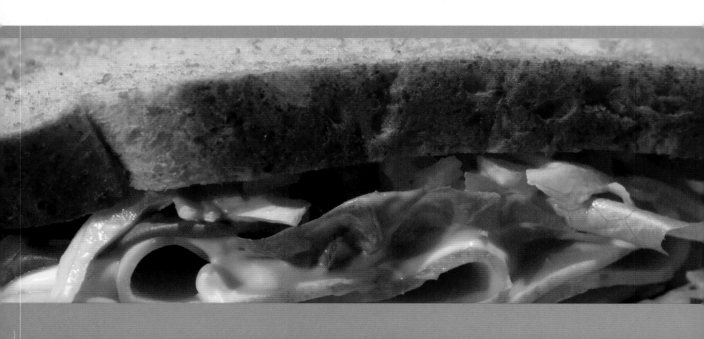

is unlikely to contain much fibre in the form of vegetables. The canned drink contains sugar, but even if it is a 'diet' drink it will contain chemicals that need to be processed by the liver, causing internal stress. The crisps contain some vitamin C, but as the potatoes have been sliced thinly and fried, those levels are likely to be low, and the fats they contain are saturated and may cause an increase in the incidence of free radicals. The sweet items obviously contain sugar.

All in all, this lunch is easy to find and satisfying in the short term, but, as well as causing blood sugar imbalances during the afternoon, its lack of vitamins C and B_5 and magnesium will exacerbate any stress that you are experiencing.

At the sandwich shop, ask for extra tomatoes in your sandwich, or try one of the many specialist soup shops that are becoming increasingly common in cities, and have vegetable soup, then a sandwich or baked potato. Do not make lunch something that you eat just to stave off hunger – it has a function, and harnessing the potential power of food can only help you.

Anti-stress foods

Choosing from the following foods at lunchtime should satisfy your hunger and supply consistent energy to see you through the afternoon, in addition to supplying the essential anti-stress nutrients (among others):

VITAMIN C FOODS	MAGNESIUM-RICH FOODS	VITAMIN B_5 FOODS
Potatoes	Almonds	Eggs
Kiwi fruit	Cod	Lentils
Broccoli	Green vegetables	Sunflower seeds
Peppers	Sunflower seeds	Soya beans
Tomatoes	Brown rice	Wholegrains
Watercress	Wholegrains	Corn

To combine these you could have an egg salad with plenty of interesting vegetables in it, as well as salad leaves. Or some fish with brown rice and plenty of delicious crisp vegetables.

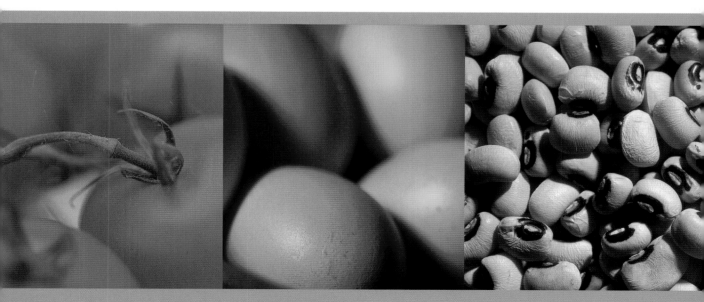

what to eat
before a night out

Evenings in a city may be spent at the theatre, the cinema, with friends in a bar or eating out. You might go to the gym, play a sport, go running or walking. You might choose to stay at home, catch up on your favourite television shows or hire a video. The choices are limitless, but often you will go straight out from work, so eating something before you leave work, or when you first meet up with friends, is important.

Assuming that you had breakfast, a mid-morning snack, lunch and an afternoon snack, all of which incorporated the principles of the City Plan, by the time you leave work you should be almost ready for something else to eat.

If you are planning to go for a drink, then having something small to eat before you set off could help to reduce the negative effects of alcohol. It might also keep you from eating too many traditional bar snacks, which are often highly salted in order to create an increased thirst to encourage you to drink even more!

The French believe in taking a spoonful of olive oil before you drink alcohol, to minimize its effects, but this is unproven, although it may have some basis in fact.

Top ten evening snacks

Consider having one of the following snacks before you set out, or stopping along the way to have something quick to eat:

Blue corn chips with avocado salsa
Cottage cheese with rice cakes
Hummus with oat cakes
Bean pâté with rye toast
A palmful of mixed pumpkin, sesame and sunflower seeds
Small piece of chicken with coleslaw
Small packet of unsalted, unroasted cashew nuts or almonds
Classic City Smoothie (see p. 124)
Hard-boiled egg
Fresh fruit

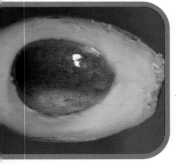

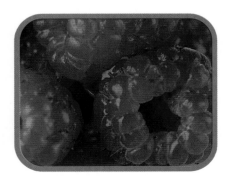

Evening meals

With the stresses that city life can bring, eating in the evenings is an excellent chance to relax and enjoy food with friends and family. Whether you sit down to an evening meal with your children, go out with friends or watch television or listen to the radio by yourself, you can make excellent food choices that promote health and will maintain your weight.

By the time evening comes, you may be tired after a busy day or a crowded journey home. Hopefully you will have eaten in line with the principles of the City Plan, so you should not be extremely hungry by the time dinner is being prepared.

The evenings are the most likely time when excess carbohydrates (those with a high glycaemic value) are stored away in fat deposits. For this reason you might want to consider reducing your carbohydrate intake in the evenings. So, rather than eating a bowl of pasta with a shop-bought sauce, you might have a few strands of pasta or rice on your plate with a good protein source, such as fish, beans, eggs or tofu, together with some broccoli, cauliflower and runner beans, thus ensuring that your evening meal includes plenty of fibre.

If you are cooking at home see pp. 106–127 for some healthy recipes that contain fibre, protein and carbohydrates in a balanced way, and are also high in antioxidants and essential fats.

Top ten dinners

Here are some ideas for easy-to-prepare dinners made with everyday foods, many of which you may already have on your shopping list or in your store cupboard (or select any of the main-course recipes in Part 3):

Stir-fried chicken with vegetables and fresh
 ginger
Baked cod with fresh dill, roast vegetables
 and wild rice
Grilled salmon with mustard-mash potatoes
 and vegetables
Bean stew with brown rice
Chicken and vegetable curry
Grilled tuna, mixed rice and vegetables
Poached chicken salad with fresh basil and
 red lentils
Stir-fried prawns with shredded vegetables
Fish stew
Roast swordfish with grilled vegetables

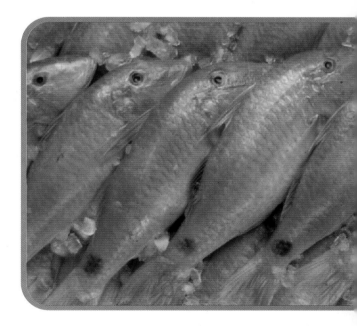

exercise time

Exercise is essential for health, yet few people realize exactly what exercise can do for them. Many people find that they avoid exercising because they feel they have not got the time or simply feel too tired. When exercise is mentioned we tend to think of the gym, but participating in a salsa dance class is exercising, as is yoga or Pilates (a form of gentle exercise that stretches and lengthens the muscles).

Types of exercise

Aerobic exercise (such as running or cycling) raises the heart beat and ideally breaks a sweat as well – this increases oxygen intake and oxygen delivery throughout the body, as the heart works harder to push the blood around the body, supplying oxygen (in addition to nutrients) and removing the natural waste products of metabolism. This type of exercise also increases the incidence of free-radical production, so the need for antioxidants is accordingly increased.

Non-aerobic exercise (such as yoga or floor stretches) is more gentle, stretching muscles and toning the body and, while you may produce a sweat, this type of exercise is not as pronounced as the aerobic alternative. It is excellent for those who do not want to 'bulk up', and prefer lean and toned muscles to the 'pumped' look.

Exercise is a vital part of this plan. Finding the time can be difficult, but it is less of a problem if you find something that you enjoy doing as you are more likely to be inspired.

Weight-bearing exercise can strengthen bones and joints, but do not think this simply means lifting weights in a gym. Lifting any weight encourages the bones to build on the opposite side of the limb. For example, lifting a weight with your hands, to build the biceps muscles, can work to strengthen the bones in your forearms. You could work out at home using a full bottle

Benefits of exercise

If undertaken regularly, which might mean twice or three times a week, exercise that raises your heart rate for more than 15 or 20 minutes can have many potential benefits. For example, it can:

Increase the levels of oxygen in the tissues

Increase cardiac output

Reduce heart rate and pulse

Reduce blood pressure

Reduce overall cholesterol levels

Help maintain and reduce body weight

Improve overall metabolic rate

Help improve bone strength

Reduce stress and improve sleep patterns

of water, or invest in some tie-on light weights, which – when attached to the ankles or wrists – increase the resistance, so making the exercise more effective. This type of activity exercises muscles more intensely and increases the efficiency of your exertions. Such exercise should not be performed quickly or jerkily, but slowly and with thought and some precision.

Finding time

Following the City Plan should have focused your mind on what you have been eating, and your diet will hopefully now include a greater proportion of fresh fruit, vegetables, wholegrains, nuts and seeds and first-class protein. You should also have reduced your intake of sugars, carbohydrates eaten on their own, tea, coffee, carbonated drinks and red meats. So now is the time to turn to exercise.

Many people do not like gyms, but there are a number of alternatives such as cycling, rowing or fast walking. Exercising with a friend or a colleague is a great way to keep up a good routine.

Exercise increases the body's metabolic rate and will therefore increase the incidence of free radicals (which are a by-product of metabolism), so anyone who exercises should ensure that they supply the body with plenty of antioxidant compounds (see p. 39). If you have done this, then your energy levels are likely to be greater than they were, leaving you with less fatigue and a greater desire to exercise. Finding the time is now your only hurdle and, given the many advantages that exercise can offer, this should be an easy task.

If you work full time, you could exercise first thing in the morning, at lunchtime or after work. Let's look at the pros and cons of each; then we will look at exercising if your time is rather more flexible.

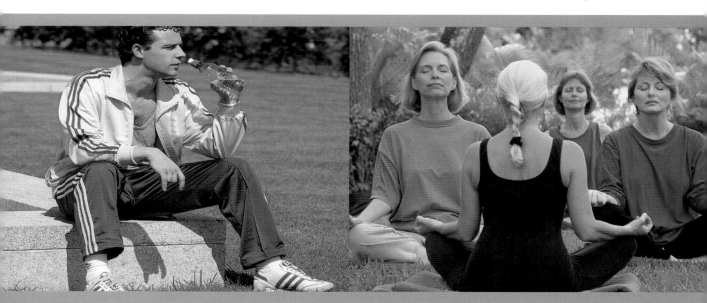

when to exercise

If you exercise in the morning you have the advantage of knowing that by the time your day begins your exercise has been done. It is also more in keeping with the body's natural production of the steroid hormone cortisol, which is higher in the mornings. Early-morning exercise is easier in the summer when the light makes it more conducive to get out of bed and get moving, so take advantage of this time and try to get outside to exercise during the summer months.

Exercising at lunchtime is a good way of breaking up the working day, as long as you do not do it on a full stomach or skip lunch altogether in order to fit your exercise routine in.

Exercising in the evenings is more practical for many people, although a busy day or general fatigue may mean that, despite leaving home with a bag packed with exercise clothes and good intentions, the bag remains unopened, for by the time work is done, exercise is a less attractive option than relaxing. However, exercising in the evenings can influence the levels of cortisol produced by the body. The natural rhythm is for cortisol levels to decrease in the evenings, in order to allow sleep, but exercise can raise levels, possibly leading to insomnia.

If you do not have to go to work and can exercise when it suits you, then exercising in the morning is preferable. However, the best time to exercise is whenever you can, and when it fits into your day. If you plan to exercise only in the mornings and you oversleep, or your commitments preclude you from getting to a class or the local swimming pool, then schedule it for later in the day when you are more likely to actually do it.

Food and exercise

Eating before exercising can reduce the potential body-fat loss, as you will be using the food you have just eaten – rather than body fat – for energy. If you get out of bed and leave the house to exercise on an empty stomach, some health professionals claim you are likely to lose more body fat, as it is this that is broken down to provide you with energy. If you do choose to eat before exercise, it is important to include some protein (as this increases muscle) and some complex carbohydrates (as these provide good, fast-acting energy).

An ideal pre-exercise snack would include some fruit or vegetables (preferably raw), some wholegrains to provide complex carbohydrates and some protein. You might choose oat cakes with hummus; an apple and some grapes with some fresh nuts; rice cakes and cottage cheese; or a pasta salad containing chicken and vegetables.

Many professional trainers believe that whatever you eat after exercise will not lead to any weight gain. This may well be true, because if you have exercised efficiently your metabolic rate will be raised, leading to greater amounts of food being used as fuel, and less as storage. Yet again, the best foods to eat are fruit and vegetables for their antioxidant properties and fibre content. Always replace lost water after exercise by drinking still mineral water at just below room temperature.

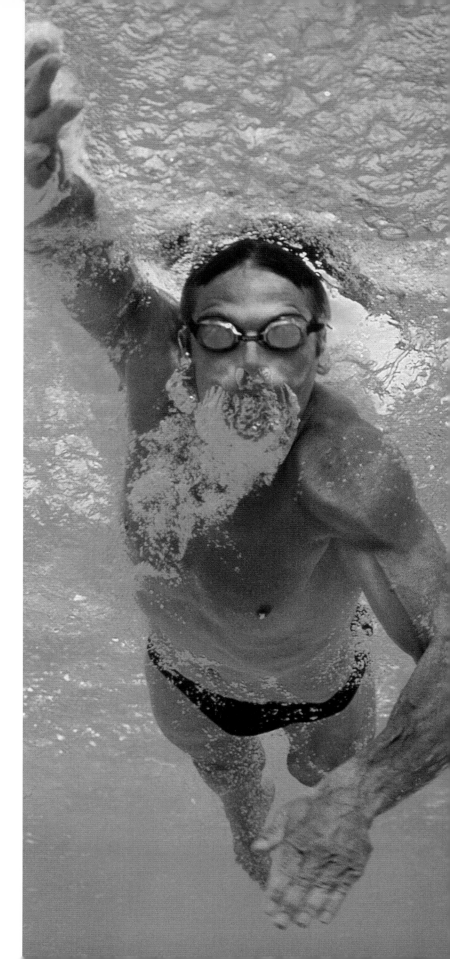

Choosing your exercise

Exercise is so varied in the types on offer that there is something to suit almost everyone. For example, if you want a strenuous aerobic workout, then running, jogging, cycling, trampolining, aerobics or step classes would all be ideal. For those who prefer more gentle, non-aerobic stretching exercise, then ballet, yoga or Pilates would be a good choice. Swimming is another form of aerobic exercise, but because it is not a high-impact activity (like running) it is particularly good for those with joint problems and the elderly, for pregnant women and those who are overweight. It also builds up stamina, strengthens and tones the muscles and promotes the circulation of lymph through the body.

Do not be limited in your choice of exercise – try as many different options as you can. Exercising just three times a week can benefit your cardio-vascular system, help you maintain your weight, and provide some valuable time to yourself, away from other commitments.

sample exercise
plan for one week

The type of exercise that you enjoy will obviously influence what you decide to do, but do not feel that you have to be tied to the gym in order to exercise. Nor does exercise have to be expensive or strenuous.

You could exercise at home, in the park or in your garden. You could check out your local community centre, because many offer classes in aerobics or step, jazzercise (a popular combination of dancing and more precise aerobic movement done to jazz music) or yoga. Local swimming baths are usually open at times to suit early-morning swims. The important thing is to do something that you enjoy.

Try to vary your programme so that you include some aerobic exercise, some weight-bearing exercise and some more gentle and meditative exercise, such as yoga. Start off gently and gradually increase the amount of exercise you do, but stop at once and seek medical advice if you get dizzy or feel a pain in your chest. Have a check-up from your health practitioner before starting an exercise routine if you are over 40 years of age, or have a medical history that includes heart or bone disease, high blood pressure or diabetes.

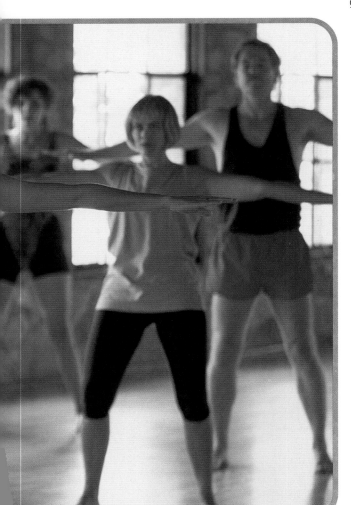

Street exercise

If you choose to run or jog along the city's streets, remember that as a natural part of aerobic exercise you will breathe more deeply, encouraging increased levels of toxins to be inhaled. A positive way to reduce this would be to avoid busy streets and head for an open space, using quiet roads that are as traffic-free as you can find. Try jogging early in the morning before the rush hour to avoid high levels of traffic fumes.

Walking is also excellent exercise, as you can vary your pace according to your fitness. The general rule of thumb is that you should walk no faster than a level at which you can still hold a conversation. This will keep your heart rate at an optimum level and should work well for most amateurs.

Sample week

Monday
At lunchtime go to a jazzercise or similar dance-based class to lift your spirits and have some fun, while simultaneously raising your heart rate.

Tuesday
Walk part of the way to or from work or going shopping, or take/collect the children from school on foot.

Wednesday
Choose from the following:

1 Rise early and do some gentle weights and 15 minutes' cycling at the gym before your daily round begins.

2 After work or your day is done, go to the gym (see 1 above) or attend a salsa lesson. Get your heart pumping and release the endorphins that can lift your mood.

3 Cycle to and from work, shopping or school, taking the long route to maximize potential benefits.

4 At lunchtime arrange to attend a lunchtime aerobic or step class with a colleague or a friend. If there is no gym nearby, then run together in the park or the nearest open space.

Thursday
Take the day off from exercise, but enjoy some gentle stretching in the morning to improve muscle tone and ease your joints.

Friday
Grasp the opportunity to exercise in the morning, perhaps choosing yoga or Pilates – both provide excellent exercise with toning techniques that will add suppleness to the joints and will work muscles without being overly strenuous.

Saturday
Exercise at leisure, perhaps in the late morning. Do this with friends and go for lunch afterwards, as by this stage of the week you deserve it.

Sunday
Once again, take a well-earned break and look forward to the week's exercise ahead.

finding peace
in the city

Noise levels can be so consistent in a city that some noises, such as the hum of traffic or aeroplanes overhead, are almost continuous – so much so that we hardly recognize they are there until they have stopped, because we have learnt not to hear them. Many people who live near railway lines simply do not notice the rumbling trains after a few days, yet visitors are acutely aware of them. This is an example of how we learn to cope with stress: the body adapts as required. This does not mean that the constant noise levels in a city become any less stressful after a while – simply that, at a conscious level, we are no longer aware of them. But hearing problems attributed to noise pollution have increased by 14 per cent since 1971 and the trend looks like continuing.

Noise levels

There are different guidelines for different noise levels, and the average length of time that we can listen to loud noise before sustaining permanent damage to our hearing varies from 16 hours for noise at 80 decibels to less than 10 minutes for noise at 115 decibels. To give you an idea of what level of decibel is emitted by familiar day-to-day occurrences, a nightclub in full swing will have music of around 100 decibels (or more), while a Boeing 747-100 taking off emits around the same level. Many cities have regular air traffic overhead and even the noise from a plane coming in to land can reach 80 decibels or so. Modern aeroplanes at least tend to be quieter than earlier versions – the latest Boeing 747-400 is 20 per cent quieter than its 1970s' predecessor.

Continuous noise causes stress and, as we know, stress leads to the release of adrenaline and to increased cortisol production. This has many effects on the body (for more information see p. 12).

Escaping noise

It is therefore important to try to find some peace and quiet away from noise, from other people, and even away from your family from time to time. This does not necessarily have to mean a place of silence and meditation, just somewhere that you find tranquil. Perhaps you have a favourite view in your city that touches you – say, a fountain in a park – or maybe you like to sit quietly in a church or other place of worship. You might want to take a detour on your journey to work and sit for a few minutes somewhere that you enjoy being.

Whatever you find peaceful, taking a few minutes out of your day to nourish your soul can only help your body to relax, relieving stress and releasing beneficial endorphins – hormones that are associated with happiness – from the brain. The possibilities are endless, and personal to you – value your private time and notice the benefits that you feel.

Sound levels in decibels

180	Rocket engine
120	Thunderclap
120	Nightclub (standing 3ft/1m in front of a loudspeaker)
100	Nightclub (standing further away from the speakers)
100	Pneumatic drill at 16ft/5m
100	Boeing 747-100 taking off (heard from inside an airport)
90	Heavy-goods vehicle (from the pavement)
85	Police siren
80	Boeing 747-400 landing (from below the flight path)
80	Personal stereo played just below full volume
80	Washing machine in a spin cycle
70	Vacuum cleaner (from 10ft/3m)
70	Telephone ringing (from 7ft/2m)
60	Ordinary conversation
50	Light traffic noise
50	Boiling kettle (from $1\frac{1}{2}$ft/0.5m)
40	Household refrigerator (from 7ft/2m)
40	Quiet office; average living-room noise
30	Soft whisper; library
10	Leaves rustling
0	Threshold of hearing

Take a moment and listen to the sounds around you. We are so familiar with noise pollution that for the most part we do not even register many of the intrusive sounds that we hear every day.

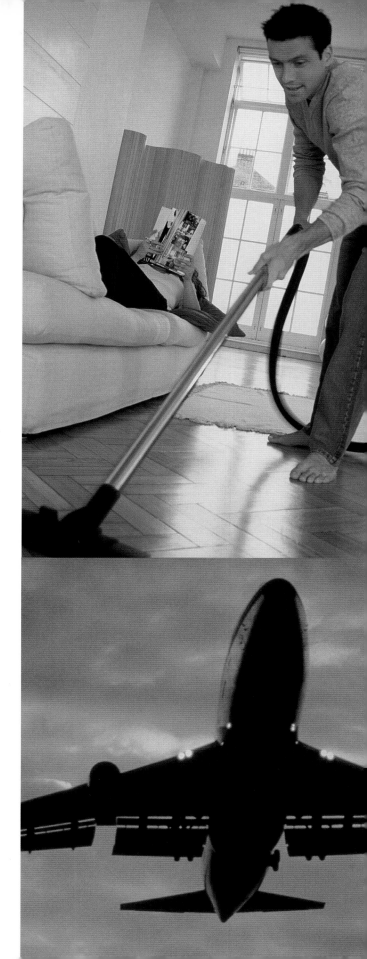

planning quiet time

In the rush of the city, quiet time has taken on added importance, and many of us get through a whole week longing for the weekend to come round so that we can relax a little.

Planning some relaxation time during the week has many potential benefits, not least in relieving stress. Quiet time really needs to make up a proportion of each day, and sometimes this requires a bit of forward planning.

As well as arranging to go for a walk with friends or alone, or taking time out from your day to sit in the park, by a fountain or in a museum, many foods can actually help the body to unwind. For instance, foods that are easily digested, such as magnesium-rich foods, encourage the muscles to relax. Including these foods in your daily diet can potentially reduce the effects of stress and calm the body. Other foods are known to have an excitatory effect on the body and should be limited as far as possible (see chart below).

Aromatherapy

Many essential oils, which are extracted from the roots, leaves, flowers, fruit, stems and bark of plants and trees, have also been found to help the body relax – calming oils include bergamot, lavender and marjoram. Either mix a few drops of essential oil with a base oil (such as almond oil) and then massage it into the skin, or add a few drops to your bath water and luxuriate in it for as long as you can spare. Alternatively, put a couple of drops of essential oil on your pillow or handkerchief. Never put pure essential oils directly on the skin, as they can cause irritation in sensitive individuals.

You could invest in an oil burner for the workplace or home. Adding a few drops of essential oil to water and warming the water over a small candle or nightlight releases the aroma into the

Foods that excite	Foods that calm
Coffee	Lentils
Tea	Brown rice
Refined sugar	Green vegetables
Salt	Citrus fruit
Cayenne pepper	Pulses
Curry powder	Tofu/soya beans
Caffeine	Camomile tea
Tobacco	
Alcohol	

air, which can act to soothe you or to excite the senses – depending on the oils that you choose
– so that you feel more able to work.

Meditation and visualization

In recent years the philosophy of the East has become more widely acknowledged and it may
help you make the most of your quiet time. Meditation was once seen as part of the 'hippie'
culture, but with the stresses of city life many people are now turning to this ancient form of
relaxation – so instead of evenings spent in a smoky bar or club, why not check out meditation
classes? They are plentiful in almost every city in the world, and are generally inexpensive,
with many potential health and psychological benefits.

Many people find meditation an excellent way to find some peace, allowing the body a chance to relax, easing digestion, boosting the immune system and improving mood and outlook.

If meditation itself does not appeal, then you could try some simple visualization techniques,
either at home or at work. Try this easy experiment if you are having a particularly busy day,
with many commitments and chores to perform. Take five minutes off and sit quietly, thinking
about a place you have visited and that you enjoyed. Perhaps it is a white sandy beach, or a
mountaintop with beautiful views – anywhere you feel is special to you. Concentrate on this
place, imagine the breeze on your skin or the sun on the sand, and visualize yourself walking
or lying on the sand or grass. After just a few minutes you may find that your day seems less
pressured and you feel more capable of coping with whatever it throws at you.

Yoga and music are other good aids to relaxation, since they encourage us to focus on them,
forgetting the troubles of the day.

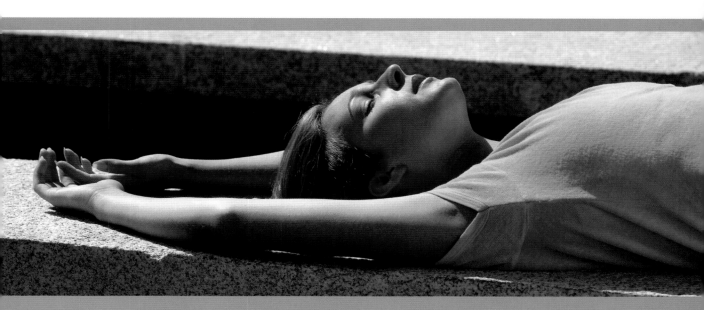

looking good

We all want to look good, and living in a city can mean that we feel added pressure to look our best. This might mean that you spend a reasonably high proportion of your income on your appearance – from your clothing to your hair. But the quality of our skin, hair and nails is profoundly affected by what we eat.

How detoxifying benefits the skin

As we have seen, detoxifying requires the release of stored toxins for processing by the liver (see p. 18). When you undertake a detox programme, it is likely that many of the toxins to which you have been exposed will be released. Unless your liver is in prime condition and your levels of stored toxins are low, the excess toxins can exit the body through the skin.

In the short term this may result in pimples, spots, blemishes and a generally poor skin tone, so if you are thinking about undertaking a detoxifying programme, choose a time when you can hibernate for a while. In Part 3 there are some excellent tips for a weekend detox plan (see pp. 133–135).

After the first two days or so your body will release the stored toxins and your liver will be working hard to eliminate them. Ensure that you eat plenty of fibre at this stage to increase excretion of the toxins from the bowel – the best sources of fibre are fresh fruit and raw vegetables, in addition to wheat bran and wholemeal bread (preferably organic, as it contains few chemicals that might hinder the process by adding further burdens to the liver).

Once the early stages of the detox programme have passed, you should begin to see the benefits in the form of clearer and younger-looking skin, brighter whites of the eyes, stronger nails and an overall improvement in your looks. But the greatest potential benefit is a general feeling of well-being, which contributes to vitality and energy.

The quality of the skin, hair and nails is an excellent barometer of the internal state of the body. For example, dull lifeless hair can often be attributed to a lack of the essential fatty acids found in fish and raw nuts. The skin also benefits from these fats, as well as from vitamin C and antioxidants. The state of the nails is particularly useful for indicating internal imbalances.

Nail health

Problem	Possible causes
White marks under the nails	Zinc deficiency
Thin, spoon-shaped nails	Vitamin B_{12} deficiency
Bumps on the nail surface	Inflammation in the body
Brittle nails that break easily	Lack of essential fats or iron
Vertical ridges on the nails	Lack of the B vitamins
Horizontal ridges	Stress or infections

Beneficial foods

Many foods can assist not only in detoxification but also in improving the quality and physical appearance of the skin, hair and nails. Here are some examples:

FOOD	CONTAINS	ASSISTS
Broccoli	Vitamin C	Collagen structure in the skin (collagen being the main protein constituent of all connective tissue); high fibre content helps eliminate toxins.
Salmon	Essential fats and vitamin E	Protection of skin from free radicals; helps skin to look plump and moist
Apples	Vitamin C and pectin	Skin health and removal of toxins from the gut.
Oats	Fibre	Toxin elimination.
Bananas	Beta-carotene and fibre	Skin integrity and toxin removal.
Molasses	Calcium	Nail growth.
Mackerel	Essential fats and vitamin D	Skin and hair quality, healthy nail formation.

Foods to avoid

Many foods and drinks can have a negative effect on your outward appearance and they are often prevalent in the typical diet of a city dweller. Avoiding the following foods can help to improve the quality of your skin, hair and nails, because they contain stimulants that may restrain important nutrients, or they inhibit absorption or stress the liver so that the daily detoxifying process is hindered:

Caffeine
Carbonated drinks
Saturated fats found in dairy
    products and red meat
Fried foods
Tobacco
Alcohol
Refined sugar

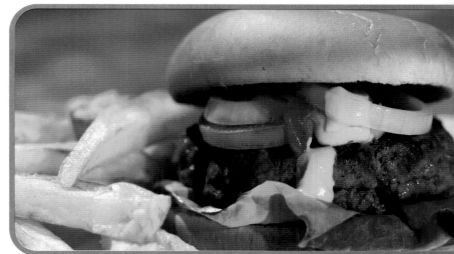

water

The benefits of water cannot be overstated. Water in abundance is essential for the health of the whole body, and not least for the appearance of the skin – if you deprive it of water, skin will become dry and flaky, but if you nourish it with water, it will bloom.

Vitamin E works in the skin to retain moisture, but we have to ensure that we are well hydrated in order for there to be sufficient water levels in the skin. The body will use the water it requires first, but many health experts believe that the skin benefits from whatever is left over.

We need to drink at least $2^1/_2$pt/1.5l of water each day – ideally plain, still mineral water (sparkling water is not taken up by the body as well as still water). The water should be drunk at just below room temperature, not straight from the fridge, because again this encourages uptake. Do not worry, however, if you only like ice-cold water, as it is better to drink it the way you like it than not at all.

Coffee, tea and carbonated drinks are not good sources of water, for they contain many other substances that can negate the positive properties of the water, in addition to having dehydrating effects of their own. This highlights the need for good quality, fresh unadulterated water.

Water is also prevalent in all fruit and vegetables, in a form that is effectively distilled, so eating an abundance of fresh produce will enhance your water intake. But do not rely on produce alone to provide water – make sure that you drink your minimum $2^1/_2$pt/1.5l daily. The results will soon be apparent in healthier-looking (and -feeling) skin.

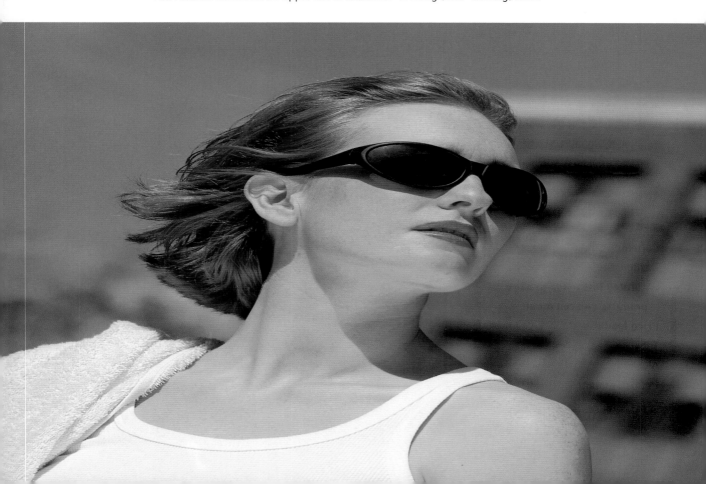

Combating dry skin

If you have dry skin this can often be attributable to a simple lack of water intake, together with a low level of the essential fats found in oils, fish and some vegetables and fruit. Dry skin can easily show the signs of ageing, as it lacks the plumpness that we associate with youthful skin.

Dry skin may also be a visible sign of a lack of vitamin A and the B group, so increasing the amount of brightly coloured red and yellow vegetables and fruits – which are rich in vitamin A and beta-carotene (the precursor of vitamin A, which is converted on the wall of the intestine) – along with wholegrains and green leafy vegetables is a good way to address this.

Zinc is also essential, as it is necessary for the optimum functioning of the sebaceous glands, which produce oil in the skin. Zinc is found in eggs, wholegrains, soya and chicken. However, if you have had dry skin for some time you may wish to consider a course of zinc supplementation (no more than 50mg from all sources, so check to see how much is contained in any other supplements you are already taking, then add in whatever is missing). There are many forms of zinc, and the citrate or liquid forms are both highly absorbable.

Foods that can contribute to dry skin are those that are high in salt, sugar and saturated fats. Excess salt interferes with the pump that allows nutrients into (and waste out of) every cell, while sugar and saturated fats affect gut health, which has a direct link to skin and general well-being. Processed foods and ready meals can often be sources of these elements, so try to eat fresh foods whenever possible, including a high proportion of raw fruit and vegetables.

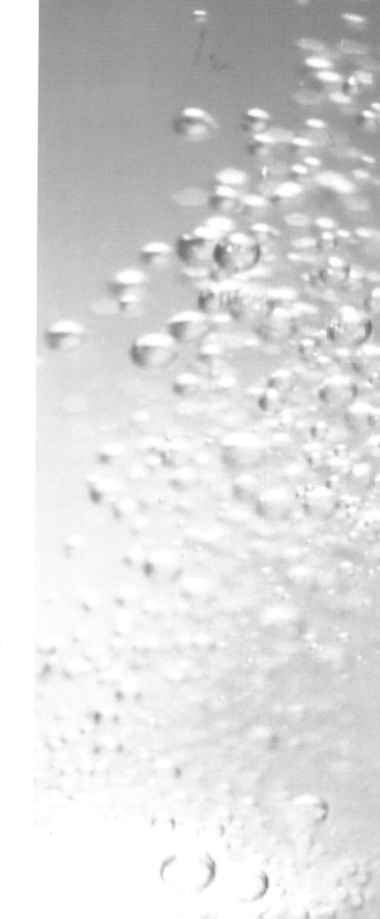

anti-ageing measures

Having seen how damaging free radicals need to be matched by healthy levels of antioxidants (see pp. 14–19), you should now be more aware than ever of how important these substances are in fighting not only disease but also the visible signs of ageing.

The process of ageing could be seen as cumulative damage caused by the incidence of free radicals which are not matched by antioxidants in the body. Few places in the body show the signs of ageing as readily as the skin, and particularly exposed areas of the body – that is, the face, neck and hands – which are more vulnerable to free-radical damage as they are often in direct sunlight. Combating ageing should always include wearing some sort of sunscreen. Most skin moisturizers now contain a sun-protection factor and should be applied daily, even in winter.

Working from the inside, however, the skin requires certain elements to maintain its structure. The most important is vitamin C, followed closely by essential fatty acids, vitamin A, the B group of vitamins, vitamin E and zinc.

The value of dark fruit and vegetables

It is interesting to note that in the same way that some people's skins are darker than others, according to their origins, so some fruit and vegetables have developed their darker colour for the same reason – as protection against the sun and as a way of using the heat and energy found in sunlight to their advantage. Compare a typical Mediterranean skin to a Nordic skin. The darker, or olive, skin has occurred over many thousands of years of evolution to suit the local environment and climate. The Nordic skin has not had to alter in the same way to cope with high levels of sunlight, and so it remains lighter in colour.

It seems that nature provides us with increased sources of protection to suit the climate in which we live. The darker varieties of fruit and vegetables are often native to warmer countries – thus the greater the risk of experiencing free-radical damage, the greater the potential source of antioxidants to match them. So to have a high level of antioxidants in the diet it is important to concentrate on the darker fruits and vegetables.

As with all areas of nutrition, just as some foods can enhance, so others can hinder. Foodstuffs that can have a negative effect on the appearance of the skin, hair and nails – even the brightness of the whites of the eyes – include all the usual suspects (see p. 81).

Beauty foods

Bearing in mind that looks come from the inside, the foods that can enhance your appearance need to incorporate as many of the following qualities as possible: antioxidant; antibacterial; fibre to clear toxins; essential fats to support skin, hair, nails and metabolism; low in saturated fats; and low in sugar.

The foods that contain most of these properties are fresh fruit and vegetables, wholegrains, fish, pulses, nuts and seeds. The familiar rule of five pieces of fruit and vegetables a day still holds true, but if you want to enhance your appearance, then eating as many beauty foods as is practical should deliver larger amounts of the essential nutrients that have anti-ageing influences, thus maximizing your looks.

Top 50 beauty foods

NUTRIENTS	FOUND IN
Vitamin A and beta-carotene	Apricots, liver, mustard greens, pumpkin, cantaloupe melon, carrots, eggs, dark-green lettuce, watercress and red peppers.
Vitamin C	Peppers, kiwi fruit, potatoes, blackcurrants, tomatoes, sprouted seeds, sweet potatoes, broccoli, papaya and citrus fruit.
Vitamin E	Eggs, almonds, hazelnuts, sunflower seeds and oil, walnuts, avocado, wheatgerm, olive oil and oatmeal.
Selenium	Tuna, molasses, mushrooms, cabbage, eggs, liver, most seafood, onions, chicken and Brazil nuts.
Zinc	Sardines, chicken, cucumber, eggs, tuna, potatoes, cauliflower, carrots, oats and almonds.

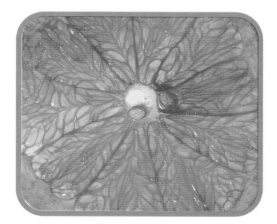

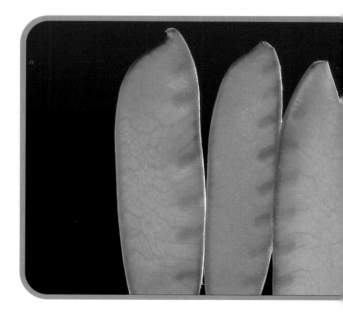

the effects of tea, coffee
and other stimulants

Many of us have come to rely unwittingly on stimulants such as tea, coffee, sugar and alcohol to see us through the day and give us a boost when needed. Such stimulants may provide some short-term benefit, but after a while these 'benefits' are barely noticed, although we still continue to crave the stimulants. A healthy liver can take up to 24 hours to process the caffeine in two cups of coffee, three cups of tea or two cans of carbonated drinks. If you drink more than that, or have strong tea or coffee every day, your liver is at risk of being overburdened, reducing its overall ability to process other toxins and in time possibly leading to increased stores of toxins.

But what effect do the individual stimulants actually have on the body?

Alcohol and refined sugars

These stimulants can alter the balance of bacteria in the colon, creating internal toxins that may be excreted through the skin. Alcohol needs to be broken down by the liver, so regular alcohol consumption can compromise liver function, creating a situation in which toxins that cannot be processed by the liver are stored in the cells. A compromised liver can also play a role in food intolerance (see p. 16 for information on increased gut permeability).

Refined sugars also play havoc with blood sugar regulation, as they cause a sharp rise in energy, which is short-lived and will probably be followed by a slump (see p. 50). This can encourage further reliance on stimulants, as the fatigue and lethargy that result are debilitating, so we turn to stimulants again for another energy boost.

Sugar – be it in alcohol, tea, coffee or carbonated drinks – also depletes magnesium levels, which can upset the stress mechanism. Magnesium plays an essential role in many processes, such as cell replication, relaxation of muscles (including the heart muscle), transmission of nerve impulses and energy production. A diet high in sugar can have a negative effect on one, or all, of these processes.

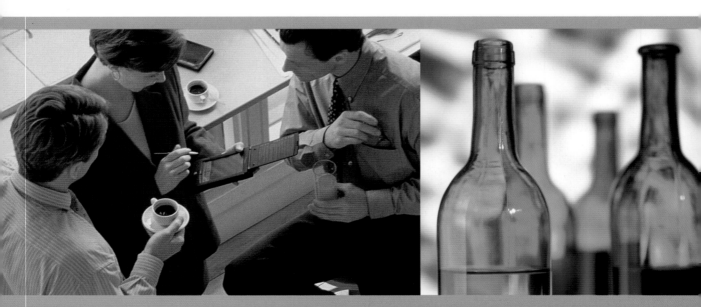

Tobacco

Smoking depletes vitamin C levels, which are essential for maintaining the collagen structure of the skin. It has long been acknowledged that smoking is carcinogenic – lung cancer is one of the most prevalent forms of cancer, and many other forms have also been linked to cigarette smoking. Smoking can also inhibit the functioning of some types of immune cells, which may lead to an increase in the incidence of colds and infections. It can also cause irritation of the digestive tract, which may reduce the levels of hydrochloric acid produced in the stomach, thereby reducing the breakdown of food and release of the nutrients contained therein.

Processed foods

Processed foods often lack the fibre that is required for efficient bowel and toxin clearance. They also contain preservatives, which are generally chemical-based, requiring processing by the liver and so adding strain to an already overworked organ. Such foods have, by their very nature, been altered from their original state by cooking or by generally changing their constituents, and more often than not this depletes their mineral and vitamin status.

Carbonated drinks

Fizzy drinks place an extra burden on the liver, as the majority of them contain chemicals that require detoxification, plus caffeine and either sugar or artificial sweeteners. They can alter the bacteria balance in the gut and reduce levels of hydrochloric acid in the stomach, thereby limiting its digestive ability and the levels of nutrients that are released from the food we eat. The phosphoric acid in carbonated drinks can also deplete essential bone nutrients, which may increase the risk of osteoporosis.

Tea and coffee

Both drinks act as anti-nutrients since they contain caffeine and tannins, which are believed to inhibit nutrient absorption and may therefore have far-reaching effects on all bodily functions. If antioxidant absorption is reduced, then the body becomes more vulnerable to the action of free radicals, and conditions associated with these rogue biochemical substances range from cardiovascular disease to the visible signs of ageing. For more on the effects of caffeine see p. 57.

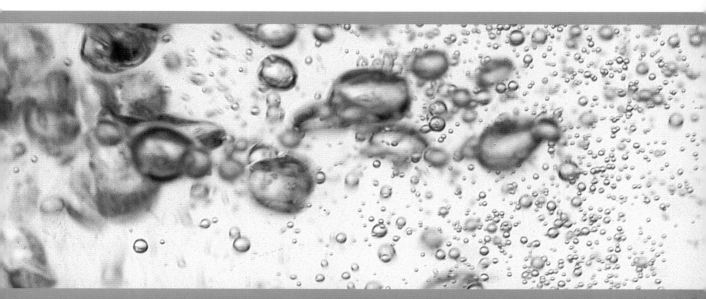

finding harmless
substitutes

There is nothing wrong in enjoying one cup of tea or coffee a day (without sugar of course), but limiting your intake or cutting them out altogether can have many potential health benefits.

Herbal teas

Herbal and fruit teas are widely available, and the combinations are exciting and full of flavour. Often drinking regular tea and coffee is done just because we want a warm drink or a break from whatever we are doing, and habit dictates that we reach for traditional choices. But herbal and fruit teas have the advantage that they offer specific benefits to the body, in terms of being calming, soothing and cleansing.

Alternative hot drinks

DRINK	BENEFITS
Apple and ginger tea	Good for stomach upsets.
Camomile tea	A calming and soothing drink.
Chicory coffee	A useful coffee-substitute, since it contains no caffeine, being made from chicory essence, not real coffee.
Cinnamon tea	Helps fight fatigue; beneficial for whenever you feel below par.
Ginger tea	Soothing for the digestive tract and extremely good for combating nausea.
Green tea	Low in caffeine, with potent antioxidant properties.
Lemon tea	Made from fresh lemon essence or leaves and hot water, this has many of the benefits of the fruit itself; not to be confused with regular black tea with a slice of lemon, which of course contains caffeine.
Lemon-balm tea	Promotes restful sleep; calming for nervous problems.
Peppermint tea	Aids the digestion of food; good for ending a meal with.

Cold drinks

Carbonated drinks are ubiquitous, and many people favour them over simple water or juice, but if you feel you must drink them, then one a day should be your limit. Some people report that they feel almost compelled to drink 'diet' drinks all day, so removing them altogether from you intake might be the best advice.

Many drinks are now marketed as 'health' drinks, but while they may contain fruit and sometimes herbs such as ginseng, they are often high in sugar. If you feel that you must drink these, then at least dilute them with 50 per cent fresh mineral water.

If your regular drink comes in a can ('diet', 'health' or otherwise), then perhaps it is time to replace these drinks with water – ideally, still mineral water.

The best drink on earth

The plain truth is that the best thing to drink is still mineral water. If you want to make it more interesting then consider adding one of the following:

Fresh lemon or lime juice
Fresh peeled ginger
Pieces of fresh fruit, such as citrus, apple or pear
Vanilla essence – two drops per $2^1/_2$pt/1.5l of water
Mint leaves
Camomile, green or herbal tea

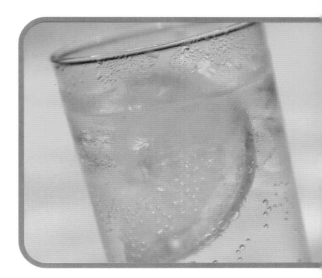

Fruit juices are a good way to get natural fruit sugars and antioxidants, and should be drunk in preference to carbonated drinks. However, they can disturb blood sugar levels, because they lack the fibre that is found in the whole fruit. Once again, the best way to drink juices is to dilute them.

Dairy drinks

While it is true that milk is a good source of calcium, it is also a source of saturated fats. Many of us were brought up believing that milk is the best source of this essential bone mineral, yet this may be attributable mostly to the power of advertising. Many vegetables, especially the darker green ones, and fresh seeds as well, contain similar levels of calcium, along with magnesium and other minerals that are used in bone manufacture and maintenance. The saturated fats in milk mean that it should be bypassed as a drink in favour of water or herbal teas, which have far more obviously beneficial effects on the body.

Yoghurt drinks are also high in saturated fats, and are more often than not sweetened with sugar or flavourings, so again they should be kept to a minimum.

recreational drugs and
their effects on the body

It is a disturbing fact that city life often involves drug use and that many people use recreational drugs regularly. The taking of drugs is in no way condoned, encouraged or approved of as part of the City Plan. We will, however, look at the most widely used drugs to see exactly what effects they have on the body, and how they can damage your health in ways that are not always publicized. All drugs increase the body's metabolic rate, thereby increasing the levels of free radicals in the body. And free radicals have been closely linked with diseases such as cardiovascular disease, cancer, arthritis and general conditions associated with ageing.

Cocaine

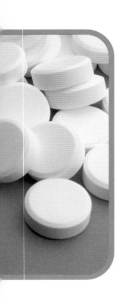

Cocaine is a substance made from leaves of the coca tree in South America. The drug is a central-nervous system stimulant that is known to heighten senses and decrease the need for sleep and food. As it works on the central nervous system, it raises the heart rate, blood pressure and breathing, through the action of adrenaline. This has many effects on the body. First, increased blood pressure and heart rate can increase the risk of cardiovascular disease. Second, adrenaline encourages the release of the hormone insulin, which can lead to internal inflammation. Furthermore, blood sugar disturbances are more likely to occur, leading to cravings – and many users misread these cravings and take more cocaine instead. As cocaine is taken through the nasal passages, problems such as nasal drip are also common.

On an emotional level, the drug is highly addictive, since many users feel that they need the drug in order to perform at work or socially. It is common for cocaine use to increase as the user becomes more tolerant to its effects on the brain, yet the physical effects of adrenaline release remain.

As the drug suppresses appetite, many people use it in an effort to lose weight. This has inherent problems, as the drug works less effectively over time and more is therefore needed. Nutrient deficiencies are common in drug users, and digestive problems are often quick to manifest themselves because the user has little or no fibre in their diet.

As cocaine is generally sold by weight, it is not uncommon for it to be mixed with other powders in order to make it last longer, or to bulk it up, and amphetamines and even talcum powder are often found in cocaine. While talcum powder may not be noxious, it was never meant to be inhaled directly into the lungs and the long-term effects of this are difficult to quantify.

One astonishing recent survey sampled 7,000 bank notes taken at random from shops and banks in London. Scientists analysed every note and found that 99 per cent contained traces of cocaine. A previous survey in Chicago some five years earlier reported that 94 per cent of notes were impregnated with the drug. This staggering statistic highlights just how prevalent the taking of cocaine has become in cities.

Ecstasy

Ecstasy is part of a group of drugs known as empathogens and is more correctly called MDMA, or methylenedioxymethamphetamine. Unlike cocaine, MDMA is a synthetic substance that is manufactured chemically, so formulas differ. Some can be considered far more dangerous than others, as 'manufacturers' can cut costs by including other substances that have no place in the body. Like all drugs, ecstasy has many potential dangers – not least addiction. Use of the drug has been shown to be harmful in pregnancy, leading to a staggering increase in birth defects of almost 3,800 per cent!

The drug works directly in the brain, blocking reabsorption of the hormone serotonin and thereby increasing the levels of circulating serotonin. Another neurotransmitter known as dopamine is also increased, as well as the hormone adrenaline. The increased serotonin levels will last for up to three hours, at which time the feelings produced by the drug will wane. Users often take another ecstasy tablet at this point in the hope of prolonging the feeling, but since serotonin levels take as long as ten days to be replenished, taking another tablet serves only to stress the liver, for no amount of ecstasy can replace the lost serotonin. The dangers of ecstasy have been well documented, and the deaths of some extremely young users have been highly publicized by the media. The drug requires breaking down in the liver, and this process can seriously affect liver function, even if no ill-effects have previously been noticed. Furthermore, as users rarely take just one tablet, the second may have few of the desired effects, only side-effects.

Because serotonin is used up by the drug, users frequently suffer from depression a few days later, often accompanied by changes in appetite and lethargy. As with cocaine, appetite suppression can lead to many potential nutrient deficiencies – not least to a shortage of those nutrients that support liver function, which is so vital for processing the drug in the first place.

MDMA increases heart rate and blood pressure, and can bring on seizures and panic attacks, feelings of paranoia and depression. Users are often encouraged to drink plenty of water while taking the drug, as it has a dehydrating effect on the body, but drinking too much water can in extreme cases lead to kidney damage, as the kidneys are placed under an enormous burden to handle large amounts of water drunk over a short time. Ecstasy also increases body temperature, yet many people find that they feel cold having taken the drug – this is attributable to MDMA's ability to interfere with the body's internal thermometer. And if the drug is mixed with alcohol, as is common in nightclubs, then the risk of liver complications is increased.

> ## Side-effects of speed
> Any of the following side-effects may be experienced as a result of taking amphetamines:
> Convulsions
> Loss of appetite
> Increased heart rate and blood pressure
> Extreme internal body-temperature fluctuations
> Insomnia
> Panic attacks
> Irritability
> Aggression
> Depression

Speed

Amphetamines, or speed, are synthetically manufactured and, like MDMA, the formulas differ, leaving room for the introduction of foreign substances. Even if the speed is untampered with, it can have many far-reaching, negative effects on the body. As with MDMA and cocaine, speed increases the levels of adrenaline in the body to abnormally high levels. In the long term this can severely damage the action of the adrenal glands, so that years after drug use has ceased complications such as insomnia, bone loss, raised blood pressure, an increased incidence of infections and irregular heart beat are not uncommon. As with all drugs, speed is illegal and the so-called 'benefits' are far outweighed by the risks, both long- and short-term.

the need for sleep

City life can mean that we are sleep-deprived. Getting out of bed early to go to work, to take the children to school or to attend classes may mean that we lose many hours' sleep every day. A recent study at the University of Chicago highlighted that people living at the beginning of the twentieth century benefited from an average of nine hours' sleep each night. In the late twentieth century this fell to just over seven hours a night.

Tests have shown that healthy adults who were deprived of sleep in research conditions found that digestion and the assimilation of carbohydrates and proteins were compromised by a lack of sleep. It could be argued that the average sleep quota of just over seven hours actually represents sleep deprivation.

Researchers also found that a lack of sleep increased signs of ageing and age-linked diseases, such as diabetes. This was attributed to the change in sleep-deprived subjects in the time that it took for them to assimilate carbohydrates into their blood sugar (see p. 50). Lack of sleep also interferes with our natural levels of hormones, such as cortisol, the stress hormone (see p. 12).

As the pressures of city life often mean that we stay out late, rise early, have busy weekends and are subject to ever-greater levels of stress, sleep and the quality of sleep that we achieve have now taken on added importance. Sleep not only gives us the chance to 'recharge our batteries', but is the time when the body sets about maintaining itself, as the growth and repair hormones take over from the activity hormones that are temporarily put out of action as we lie at rest.

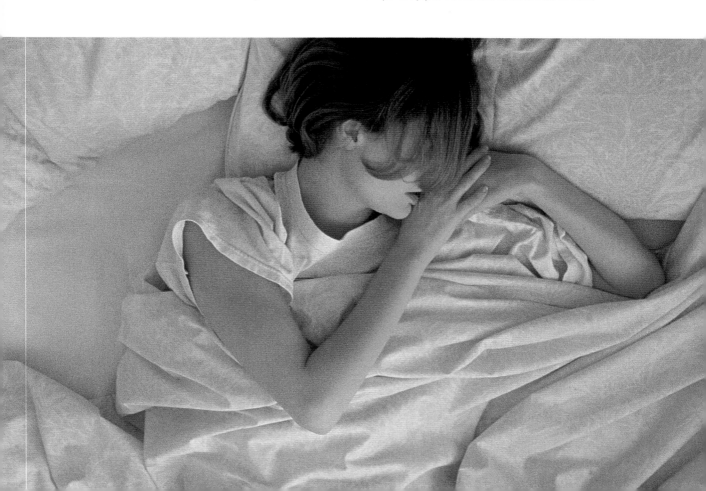

Sleep foods

There are a number of nutritional elements that can promote sleep and increase its quality. The sleep mechanism is triggered by the presence of the amino acid tryptophan. This competes with other amino acids to cross the blood-brain barrier (see p. 14), which is the layer protecting the brain from potential toxins and unwanted substances (in addition to acting as a filter for amino acids).

Eating carbohydrate-rich foods can suppress the levels of all amino acids with the exception of tryptophan – allowing it alone to cross the blood-brain barrier, thereby promoting sleep. However, if we apply the principles of efficient blood sugar management, then a carbohydrate-rich snack at bedtime could lead to sharp rises in blood sugar levels, which can promote increased fat stores. Instead, tryptophan itself is found in some foods, such as cottage cheese, bananas, dried dates, milk, peanuts and turkey. Perhaps this is why our grandmothers would have had a glass of warm milk to help them sleep.

The last point to be made here about sleep relates to stress and sugar, both of which can reduce the levels of magnesium in the body. As magnesium is responsible for the relaxation of muscles (and calcium for their contraction), including some magnesium in the evenings, perhaps in supplement form, can further promote sleep.

Bearing all these facts in mind, there are combinations of foods that can promote sleep, either because they combine carbohydrates to improve tryptophan absorption or because the foods themselves contain tryptophan.

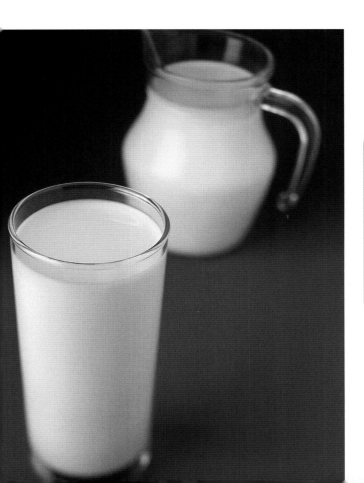

Ideal sleep foods
Banana milkshake with a little tofu blended in
Cottage cheese and oat or rice cakes
Dates and cottage cheese
Date and soya-milk smoothie
A palmful of almonds and a piece of fruit
Sunflower seeds and a banana
Rye bread with a slice of turkey
Rice cake with unsweetened nut butter

eating at the right times
to promote sleep

On the preceding pages we saw how important sleep is, as well as how potentially to improve sleep. We also saw which foods can promote improved sleep patterns. But does it matter at what times we eat? Does this affect the potential quality of our sleep?

It is well known that eating too late can inhibit sleep, because the overworking of the digestive system late at night can keep us awake. Ideally you should not eat during the hour before you go to bed.

Including some magnesium-rich foods at dinner may help to relax the muscles, promoting a feeling of calm. Many people suffer from cramped muscles during the night, and magnesium is particularly important for this group. Magnesium is also a stress mineral (see p. 31) and is required in greater amounts during times of strain. If you do feel pressurized, then the role of magnesium is even more important to you.

Balancing blood sugar levels also plays an important role in promoting sleep. Eating small, frequent meals can help to even out glucose levels in the body, so understanding the section on blood sugar management (see p. 50) is highly recommended.

Ideally, you should be eating breakfast at, say, 8 a.m., a small snack around 11 a.m., lunch at 1 p.m., another small snack at 4 p.m. and dinner at 7.30 or 8 p.m. To keep your blood sugar balanced it would be advisable to have a small snack at 11 p.m., assuming that you are planning to be asleep by midnight.

Magnesium-rich foods

The following foods are all rich sources of this vital mineral:

Cod

Halibut

Herring

Green vegetables

Nuts

Shrimp

Tofu

Swordfish

Sunflower seeds

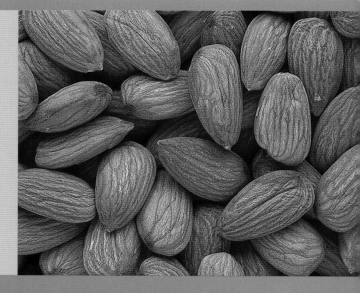

Insomnia

Everyone suffers from occasional sessions of sleeplessness and there may be many factors at play that are responsible for it, but if you experience prolonged insomnia, take a good, hard look at your nutritional status.

Hopefully you are avoiding caffeine at all times, but it is especially important to avoid it in the evenings, as it can disturb sleep patterns and blood sugar management. Replace coffee with camomile tea or, if you must, have decaffeinated coffee that has had the caffeine removed using the 'water' (rather than the 'solvent') method. Once again, refined sugar can stimulate the body, so avoid this in the evenings (but preferably at all times!). Remember that carbonated drinks contain sugar and caffeine, so they should be avoided as well, even the 'diet' or 'lite' versions, since they also contain caffeine, although the sugar has been replaced by chemical sweeteners.

Avoiding highly spiced foods could also help, as many spices are thought to have a stimulatory effect on the body. You could try replacing strong curries or hot Thai food with milder versions, or perhaps eat simpler food altogether. And make sure that you finish eating two to three hours before you intend to go to bed. You might also consider taking a magnesium supplement, but as there are many types of magnesium formula, look for one that gives you no more than 400–600mg.

If you find that you often wake up during the night, then your levels of cortisol may be rising at the incorrect times. Cortisol rises naturally in the mornings, yet long-term stress can adversely affect this. If this is a recurrent problem you may wish to work with a nutritional consultant to ascertain when your levels rise and fall – this is done by means of a simple saliva test (known as the Adrenal Stress Index or ASI).

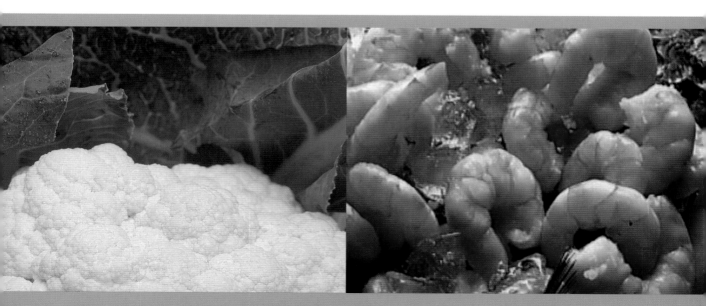

mood and depression

Depression and anxiety are becoming more common – one need only look at the profits of the drug companies that manufacture antidepressants to see how frequently these medications are being prescribed. The pressures that city life holds may be contributing to feelings of anxiety. Mood is affected by blood glucose levels, and when these are low we may feel irritable or anxious, which may be diagnosed as depression.

It is important, however, to differentiate between clinical depression and simply anxiety or 'feeling blue'. If you experience long-term unhappiness then you may be suffering from clinical depression. If that is that case, then you would be well advised to consult your health practitioner.

In recent years the chemistry of the brain has been closely researched, and it has been established that nutrition can play an important role in balancing the neurotransmitters that are involved in dictating how we feel on an emotional level.

Food groups and mood

To avoid blood sugar lows, we have already seen that we should ideally eat a combination of fibre, carbohydrates and protein at each meal or snack (see p. 50). Furthermore, we should eat almost before we truly experience hunger, so that we avoid the extreme lows that can exacerbate feelings of depression or anxiety.

However, carbohydrates must be eaten to ensure that the amino acid tryptophan is absorbed into the brain (see p. 93 for further details about how this link works). It is tryptophan that is a precursor of serotonin – a neurotransmitter that has long been associated with improving mood and outlook. Including some foods that are rich in vitamin B_6 can assist in the synthesis of serotonin, so eat avocados, carrots, hazelnuts, salmon and brown rice. Tryptophan itself can be found in bananas, turkey, cottage cheese, raw peanuts, milk and dried dates.

Allergies and mood

If you suffer from sensitivities to certain foods, this can easily affect your mood. Sufferers from full food allergies (as opposed to food intolerance, which is a milder reaction) often report that depression is part of their reaction to the food they now avoid. See p. 16 for information on gut permeability (or leaky gut syndrome), as a compromised gut lining can increase the likelihood of food sensitivities or intolerances.

The most common foods that can cause problems are wheat, dairy products and citrus fruit. It is not fully understood why wheat has the capacity to cause sensitivities, although it is likely that it is linked to the presence of gluten, which although found in oats, barley and rye, is more prevalent in wheat. Think about how often you eat wheat as it is present in a large proportion of common foods.

If you have persistent symptoms of any of the above, then you should consult your physician.

The dopamine pathway

The chemical dopamine acts like a neurotransmitter, as it assists the efficient transmission of nerve impulses, and low levels of dopamine have been linked to anxiety and depression. The use of some drugs can block the dopamine receptors in the brain – a situation that can manifest itself as increased anxiety.

Dopamine is synthesized from an amino acid called tyrosine, which can be found in protein foods such as cottage cheese, herrings, sesame and pumpkin seeds. It is also found in carbohydrate foods such as bananas and avocados. Tyrosine deficiency is rare, however, and is usually found only in those who are on a strict diet.

Tyrosine can be supplemented, and many people have had significant success in improving their mood by so doing, although this course of action should only be undertaken with supervision from an appropriate health practitioner.

Anxiety and depression are very common, and in many cases are linked in part to what is eaten. Ensuring that your brain is well supplied with nutrients, identifying possible food intolerances, and avoiding stimulants can provide relief for many people.

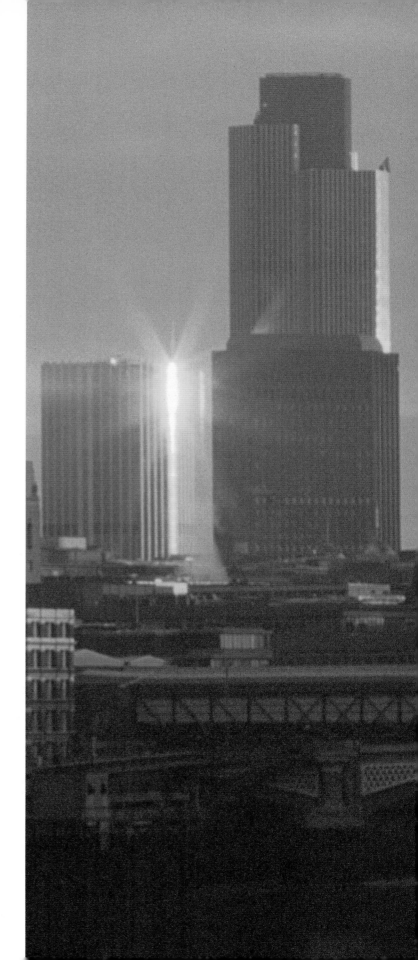

be happy

It is interesting to note that trials have identified low levels of many of the B group of vitamins in those people who are suffering from depression. Increasing your intake of foods that contain these vitamins can often assist in alleviating cases of mild depression – a simple remedy that you can put into action yourself, without the need to visit your health practitioner.

The vital B vitamins

VITAMIN	ALSO KNOWN AS	FOUND IN
B_1	Thiamine	Brewer's yeast, brown rice, wheat germ, soya beans.
B_3	Niacin or niacinamide	Fish, eggs, brewer's yeast, wholegrains, poultry.
B_{12}	Cyanocobalamin	Fish and dairy products; the only vegetable source is spirulina (a blue-green algae), although it is not clear whether humans can absorb the B_{12} from it.
B_9	Folic acid	Calves' liver, soya flour, green leafy vegetables, eggs, brown rice.

If you decide to supplement the B vitamins, be sure to choose a high-quality B-complex that covers the whole range of B vitamins. Side-effects are rare, as B vitamins are water-soluble so any excesses are usually excreted in the urine. However, long-term intake of some individual B vitamins is not recommended, so consult a qualified nutritionist who can devise an appropriate regime. Do not be alarmed if your urine becomes a bright yellow colour after taking a B-complex supplement – this is simply the excess B_2, or riboflavin, being excreted.

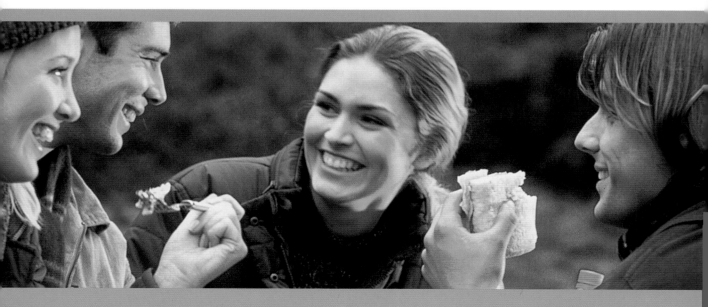

Mood and zinc

Low zinc levels have also been associated with feelings of depression, yet this link is often overlooked by the medical profession, sometimes in favour of antidepressants. Answer the questions posed in the 'zinc level test' and, if you feel that any of the symptoms relate to you, and you also suffer from depression or anxiety, you might want to consider adding some zinc rich foods to your diet. Again this is a simple remedy – as long as you keep within the recommended zinc levels – that could produce dramatic results.

If you do decide to supplement with zinc, ensure that you do not take more than 50mg daily from all sources; so if you are taking any other supplements, check the labels and add up how much zinc you are getting in total. Better still, seek the advice of a professional, who can advise you more fully.

City pollution and depression

It is known that the presence of lead in the atmosphere can contribute to feelings of depression and anxiety. As the air in the city is likely to be affected by traffic fumes, any low moods you may experience could be exacerbated by toxic metals that have entered your body. You can read more about this in the section on toxins on pp. 14–17.

The removal of toxic metals from the body requires that the liver is fully supported and that there is ample fibre in the diet to ensure that toxins are eliminated efficiently from the bowel. The antioxidant nutrients are vital for the optimum functioning of the liver, and these are found in abundance in fresh fruit and vegetables (see p. 39).

If you can help to counter any low moods that you experience by means of simple, healthy nutrition and supplementation, and can put into principle at least some of the ideas outlined in the City Plan, then you will be in a better position to enjoy life in the city to the full and to reap its rewards.

Zinc level test

Do you:

Have white marks on your fingernails?

Rarely feel hungry?

Have pale skin?

Have stretch marks around the abdomen or back?

Have oily skin, perhaps with some acne?

Experience frequent colds or flu?

Zinc rich foods

The following foods are rich in the essential mineral zinc:

Blackstrap molasses

Sesame seeds

Eggs

Turkey

Herring

Salmon

Soya products

Mackerel

Tuna

Sardines

troubleshooting

SUBJECT	AIMS	REMEDY
Food groups	The best balance	Combining protein, carbohydrates and fibre at every meal should help you balance blood glucose levels so that you feel more energetic and avoid energy slumps. Experiment with combinations, noting how you feel.
Snacks	What to eat	Snacks should be eaten in between main meals, and fruit is always an excellent fall-back. Try some of the snacks listed in the recipe section starting on p. 105.
Lack of time to shop	Easy ideas	Shop in advance – perhaps one evening or at a weekend – using the list on p. 133, which gives details of different meals to make using just 12 ingredients, and which should see you through a few days.
Breakfast	Combining foods	Combining the food groups is essential – try scrambled eggs on rye toast, oat porridge with fruit, tofu smoothies, unsweetened yoghurt and fruit salad.
Street breakfasts	Food on the run	Pass on the croissant and the coffee, and have a herbal tea and a yoghurt or sugar- and honey-free oat flapjack instead. These are less likely to affect your blood sugar levels negatively, and the oats are a good source of fibre.
Office foods	Ideas	Keep a bag of fresh, unroasted almonds and some fruit in your desk drawer, or perhaps some oat cakesand a jar of unsalted, unsweetened nut butter or an avocado.

SUBJECT	AIMS	REMEDY
Lunches	Ideas	Eat overfilled sandwiches, always with a good protein source and alternating breads whenever possible. Have a baked potato and some baked beans, or tuna, instead of sandwiches every day. Bring lunch in from home as often as possible.
Business lunches	Alternatives	Remember to combine some protein, carbohydrates and fibre, and to limit your alcohol intake. This way of eating is more likely to keep you alert and productive well into the afternoon.
Going straight out from work	Ideal foods	Have a small snack before you go out, or eat early before you start your evening. Even having a couple of pieces of fruit and some oat or rice cakes can keep you going, and will provide fibre and antioxidants that can potentially help you combat smoky atmospheres.
Exercise	Principles	Exercising every few days, even if you only manage twice a week, can help reduce cholesterol and improve concentration and oxygen uptake in the body.
Time for exercising	Suggestions	Aim to do some exercise at least three times a week. Doing exercise only at weekends is not ideal – regular exercise has more benefits, so some aerobic exercise every few days is preferable. See p. 70 for suggestions on how best to exercise, and how to fit it in even if you feel you are too busy.

Peace	Relaxing	Find some peace and quiet for yourself, every day. Take a detour on the way to work through the park, or take a moment away from your obligations and visit somewhere that you enjoy. Take the opportunity to reflect, allowing your stress mechanism some time out. Stress hormones will decrease, thereby improving sleep, mood and possibly your attitude.
Quiet time	Food suggestions	Foods that relax you include herbal teas, fruit and vegetables. Avoid caffeine and refined sugars, as these can have an excitatory influence on the body. Strong herbs and spices potentially have the same effect, so limit these if you feel at all stressed.
Looking good	Detoxifying	Undertaking a detoxification programme should allow the body to release toxins that have been stored in the tissues. Remember that you are likely to experience some minor skin problems, so drink plenty of water and eat as much raw fruit and vegetables as you can manage for their fibre and antioxidant properties.
Beauty foods	Ideas	The best foods to improve looks are those that contain vitamins A, C and E, together with the minerals selenium and zinc. Eat plenty of fresh produce, wholegrains and fresh fish, for its essential fatty acids, which can improve the look of skin, hair and nails. Avoid sugars and yeasts, as they can promote imbalances in the colon that can lead to skin and nail problems. Take a vitamin B-complex supplement daily.
Energy foods	Supplements and food ideas	For improved energy, take a high-quality B-complex supplement every day, as well as an antioxidant compound and perhaps some chromium (but no more than 400mcg a day) to help avoid cravings for sweet food. Avoid relying on caffeine and sugar for short-term energy – this is often followed by a dip in energy that can bring with it anxiety and irritability.

Tea, coffee and other stimulants	How they affect you	Frequent use of tea, coffee and carbonated drinks leads to raised blood sugar, which in turn causes the hormone insulin to be produced by the pancreas. Excess insulin has been linked to many inflammatory conditions, and in some cases can increase fat stores. Caffeine also depletes valuable minerals and B vitamins, and acts as a mild diuretic, risking dehydration.
Smoking and second-hand smoke	Warnings	Smoking has long been associated with an increased incidence of cancers, so if you can stop smoking the benefits are numerous. To help you stop smoking, learn how to balance blood sugar levels in order to avoid highs and lows, which can increase cravings for stimulants such as nicotine.
Replacing stimulants	Alternatives	Replace stimulants with herbal teas, water and diluted juices. Cut down on carbonated canned drinks and favour still mineral water when possible.
Drugs	Dangers	All recreational drugs increase adrenaline release, which exacerbates stress. Aside from being illegal, drug use is addictive and deleterious to all aspects of health.
Sleep	Sound advice	If you have trouble sleeping, avoid all stimulants throughout the day, and eat plenty of green leafy vegetables and fresh seeds, as they contain magnesium, which is involved in relaxing the muscles. Consider taking a magnesium supplement last thing at night.
Eating at the right times	When to eat	To balance blood glucose levels effectively, eat small meals – little and often is advisable. Do not allow yourself to get very hungry, as this can lead to food choices being made from a position of hunger and blood sugar lows.

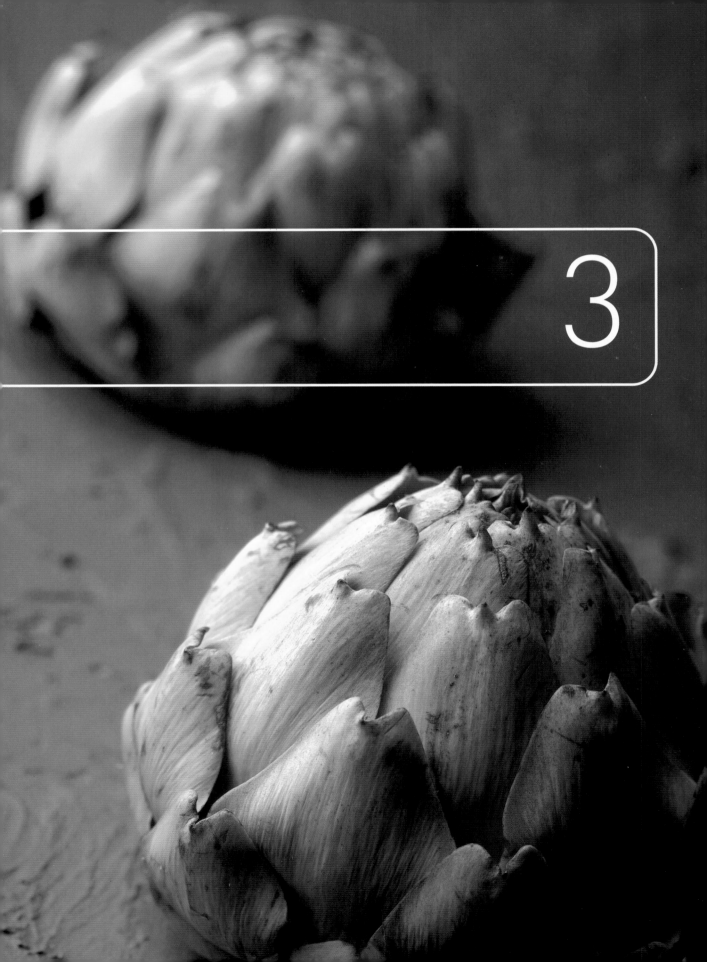

3

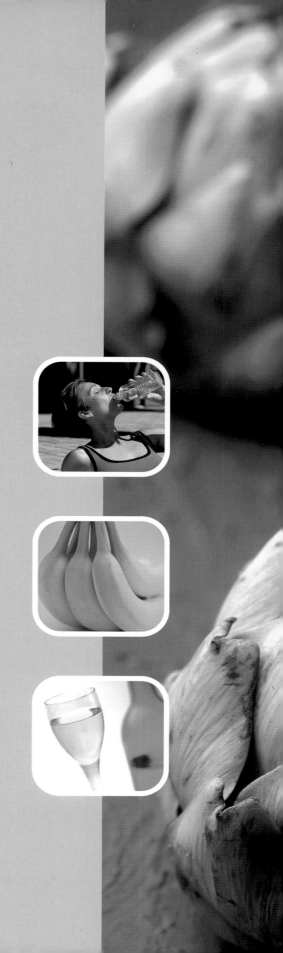

recipes
& plans

soups

Soups make a wonderful standby, and really could not be easier to make. All the soups suggested here are vegetable-based, so in eating them regularly you will be taking advantage of the whole range of nutrients that vegetables have to offer. Such soups are naturally rich in antioxidants and minerals, and low in fats.

There is always some nutrient loss when vegetables are cooked, particularly of the B group of vitamins and vitamin C. When vegetables are softened in stock to make soup, however, the liquid absorbs much of these water-soluble nutrients, and as we also consume the liquid we therefore benefit from a fair proportion of the original nutrient content.

The fibre in vegetables is broken down through cooking, so if you do eat soup regularly, remember to balance it with some vegetable-sourced fibre. For instance, have a small salad of some leaves and raw vegetables on the side.

As the soups that follow are vegetable-based, they contain no protein. If you like, you can address this by adding some cooked chicken, or even raw, cubed chicken breast, poaching it in the soup as it warms (ensure that it is properly cooked, though). Alternatively you could add cubed tofu, flaked salmon or cod for a more substantial meal, thereby adding protein as well.

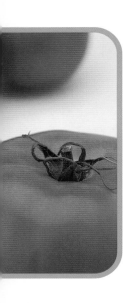

Basic Soup Recipe

This is the simplest way to make soup, and the results are excellent every time. You need two large saucepans and one wooden spoon, plus:

> 1 onion
> extra-virgin olive oil
> fresh vegetable stock (or stock powder made up with $2^1/_2$pt/1.5l water)
> vegetables of your choice, coarsely chopped

Chop the onion finely and add it to the saucepan with a little oil. Warm over a low heat, stirring with the wooden spoon, until the onions become translucent, but do not let them burn or brown too much, as this means that the oil has overheated.

If you do not have fresh vegetable stock (this can be bought at many supermarkets, but is an expensive way to get a simple stock), then boil a kettle, pour the water into the second saucepan and add in some powdered vegetable stock (this is preferable to many stock cubes, as it is yeast-free and lower in salt). Simmer until the powder has dissolved.

Add the chopped vegetables to the first saucepan, combine them with the onion, then pour in the stock. Bring slowly to the boil, then turn down the heat and cover. Leave to simmer for 20 minutes, then remove from the heat. Allow the liquid to cool, then blend it in a blender or food processor (a blender works best). Return to the saucepan, warm through and serve.

Soup suggestions

Below are some examples of vegetables that work well in soups. Choose any one of them, or experiment with combinations that appeal to you. All vegetables are rich in antioxidant nutrients, but some are believed to have other qualities that can help support the body during the particular stresses and challenges that city life brings with it.

VEGETABLE	PROPERTIES
Broccoli	Contains anti-cancerous indoles; stimulates liver function; has antibiotic and antiviral properties.
Cabbage	Stimulates the immune system; has anti-cancer properties.
Beetroot	Assists liver function; cleans the intestines.
Leek	Cleanses the digestive tract and helps eliminate toxins.
Squash	Re-alkalizes the body; rich in antioxidants.
Tomato	Rich in lycopene, a potent antioxidant.
Celery	Anti-cancerous; aids efficient digestion.
Asparagus	Stimulates kidney function; antibacterial.
Cauliflower	Anti-cancerous; helps reduce blood pressure.
Sweet potato	Relieves gut irritation; detoxifies the liver and kidneys.
Carrot	Detoxifies the colon and kidneys; antiviral and antibacterial.
Celeriac	Benefits the nervous system; also a diuretic.
Fennel	Helps digest fats.
Mushroom	Stimulates the immune function; potentially anti-cancerous.
Lentil	Provides minerals to aid muscle action.
Pea	Supports efficient liver function.
Pepper	Antioxidant and antibacterial, so it supports the immune system.
Spinach	Helps regulate blood pressure; assists the immune system in fighting infection.
Parsnip	Improves bowel function, which helps clear excess toxins and heavy metals.
Watercress	Mildly diuretic; stimulates the thyroid to increase the body's metabolic rate.

Herbs and spices for soups

Add interest to your soup by adding herbs and spices:

Coriander

Basil

Parsley

Dill

Tarragon

Cumin

Curry powder

Cardamom pods

Thyme

Bay leaves

Chives

Cayenne

Soup tips

- Freeze the onion for half an hour before you chop it, to reduce tears.
- Add half a peeled potato to thicken the soup if you prefer a more solid consistency.
- Do not add any salt, just some white pepper after cooking (white pepper works better in soup than black, as it dissolves more easily).
- Make extra soup and freeze some for later on.
- Add herbs to the stock before you blend it, for interesting flavours – but keep some for a garnish.
- Some soups, such as tomato, watercress, and leek and potato (vichyssoise), are delicious served iced in the summer.

Take Stock

City life is unlikely to afford you much time to make your own stock, so use powdered bouillon stock, or stock cubes instead, favouring the salt-free versions. Most supermarkets now sell fresh stock which is a good alternative to powdered stock. If you have time to make your own stock, simply take 2 litres of fresh water and add in 1 peeled onion, 2 carrots, 1 bay leaf, and at least 3 other types of vegetables you have to hand. Bring to the boil and simmer for 30 minutes. Leave to cool and remove the vegetables and either use the stock straightaway or freeze for later use. For a richer stock, add in some chicken bones, or whole chicken breasts, which should be discarded when the stock has cooled.

Although this is essentially not a cookbook, these recipes have been included as they incorporate the principles of the City Plan. They combine foods that are rich in antioxidants, fibre, protein and complex carbohydrates, and use ingredients that are generally available from local foodstores or markets. The recipes are easy to cook, and are suitable for families, eating alone or entertaining friends.

starters

The following starters or appetizers will give you a few ideas about how best to combine your foods. If you have a purely vegetable-based starter, then do ensure that your main course contains a little protein. If your chosen starter already contains some protein, then you could equally prepare it as a light lunch or supper, without having to have a main course in addition.

Asian Chicken Salad

Chicken is low in fat, yet high in fibre and B vitamins. Onions are known to reduce blood coagulation, while the peppers, cabbage and cucumber that this salad contains all provide fibre and are rich in antioxidant nutrients.

To make the dressing, combine the onion, rice wine, ginger, pine nuts, walnut and chilli oil, and the tamari sauce in a bowl. Leave to allow the flavours to blend together.

Poach the chicken breasts in vegetable stock over a low to medium heat for 15 minutes, then remove from the liquid and allow to cool on a plate. Cut the chicken into strips and combine in a salad bowl, or on individual plates, with the pepper, cucumber, cabbage and salad leaves.

Pour over the dressing, garnish with fresh coriander or basil leaves and serve.

Variation: tuna or salmon works well instead of the chicken, if you prefer.

$1/_3$ red onion, sliced

2 tbsp rice wine

2 tsp freshly grated ginger

4oz/100g pine nuts

3 tsp walnut oil

1 tsp chilli oil

2 tbsp tamari sauce

4 chicken breasts

$1^3/_4$pt/1l vegetable stock

1 yellow or red pepper, sliced

1 cucumber, sliced into fine strips

7oz/200g red cabbage, shredded

7oz/200g salad leaves

coriander or basil leaves to garnish

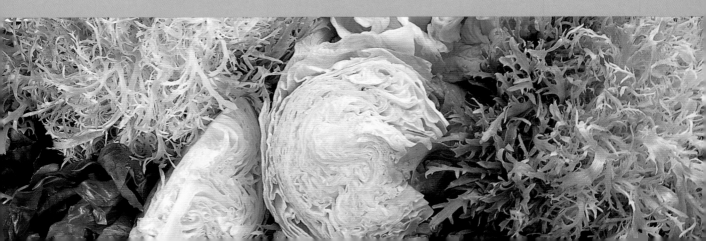

Summer Cucumber Salad

Cucumber skin contains sterols, which are a factor in reducing overall cholesterol levels. Yoghurt contains beneficial bacteria that are required in the colon to support the immune system. Lettuce contains silicon, which is supportive to the joints and connective tissue. This salad is also rich in antioxidants.

4 large cucumbers
1 large unwaxed lemon
7oz/200g plain, low-fat, bio
    unsweetened yoghurt
3 tbsp fresh dill, chopped
black pepper
4 tbsp extra-virgin olive oil
7oz/200g salad leaves

Slice the cucumber as finely as you can, or pass it through a food processor.

Chop up some lemon zest and place it in bowl with the yoghurt, the juice from half the lemon, the dill and freshly ground black pepper. Add the oil, using a fork to combine the ingredients – drizzle the oil into the bowl while combining them, as you need to create a thick consistency.

Add the cucumber and mix it in well, so that it is thoroughly covered with the dressing. Serve with salad leaves, in a bowl or on individual plates.

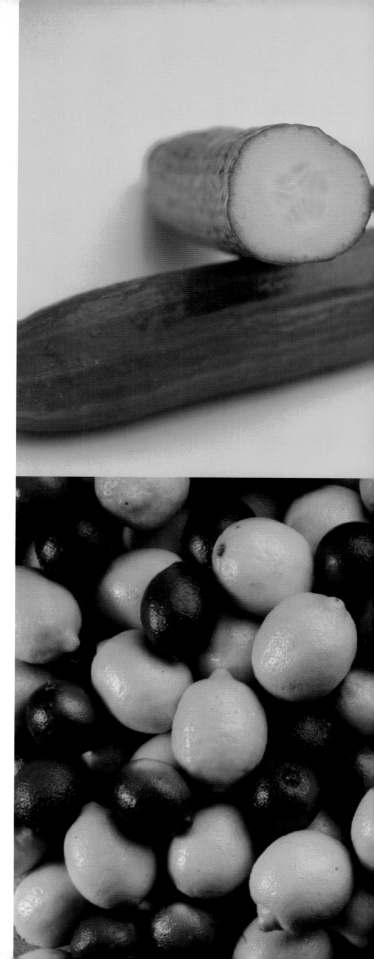

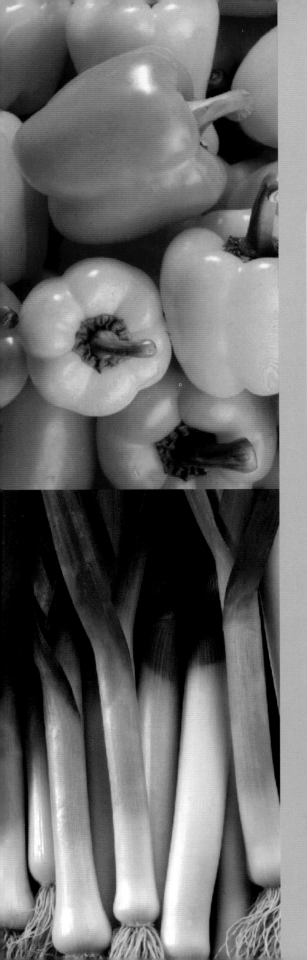

Grilled Vegetables with Parsley

This vegetable dish is rich in a wide variety of antioxidants, which can be protective against the free radicals that are involved in many degenerative diseases. In particular vitamin C, beta-carotene, selenium, zinc and calcium are all to be found in these vegetables.

1 large aubergine
1 red pepper
1 yellow pepper
1 red onion
1 white onion
1 large leek
1 head of fennel
1 clove of garlic
1 tbsp extra-virgin olive oil
black pepper
4oz/100g flat-leaf parsley, chopped

Slice all the vegetables except the garlic.

Heat some water in a large pan until it is simmering. Add the vegetables to the water for just 3 minutes. Then remove them from the water, place in a colander and run under cold water to freshen them. Pat dry on a tea towel.

Crush the garlic and combine it with a little oil and freshly ground black pepper.

Warm the grill to a medium heat (not high), then arrange the vegetables on a baking tray and drizzle a tiny amount of the seasoned oil over them. Place under the grill for approximately 7 minutes, then turn the vegetables over and repeat. Do not allow the vegetables to burn; when they start to brown, remove them from the grill or turn them over. If you do allow the vegetables to burn they may be potentially carcinogenic and should be discarded.

Serve warm, or cool if you prefer, sprinkled with the parsley for garnish.

Variation: for a treat you can also shave some Parmesan cheese over the vegetables, but be sparing – Parmesan is high in saturated fats.

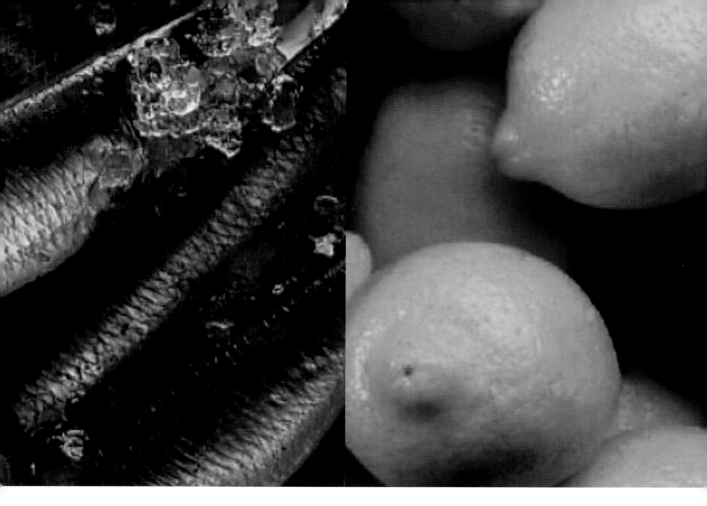

Smoked Mackerel Pâté

Mackerel contains essential omega-3 fats, which support the immune and cardiovascular systems. Cucumber and lemon are both sources of antioxidants and may have anti-cancer properties.

In a food processor add the juice from half the lemon to the chopped mackerel fillets and crème fraîche. Blend together for 1 minute for a coarse pâté, or for 2 minutes for a smoother consistency. Remove and place the pâté in a serving bowl or in individual ramekins. Then dice the cucumber and fold it in.

This pâté is excellent served on oat cakes, rye toast or on its own.

Variation: if you prefer a spicy dish, use peppered mackerel fillets instead.

1 large unwaxed lemon
4 smoked mackerel fillets
7oz/200g crème fraîche
1 large pickled cucumber

main courses

The following main courses have been designed to provide a first-class source of protein, together with fibre from vegetables. You should always try to add to these main courses by having a starter or side-dish that consists of vegetables and some complex carbohydrates – you could choose rice or pasta (but not large quantities of either) to accompany them. Recipes for vegetables and grains can be found on pp. 120–123, but do not feel that all vegetable dishes have to be complicated. Simple, steamed vegetables will complement any of the following main courses.

You do not have to follow any of the recipes to the letter. Be creative and try replacing any ingredient that you are not keen on with something that you prefer; likewise you can increase or decrease the quantities that you use to suit your own taste. The important thing is that the principles are understood and followed, and not that every individual ingredient is used.

All recipes serve four people, unless otherwise stated.

11oz/300g sweet potato (or
    celeriac)
11oz/300g salmon, poached in fish
    stock and flaked
1 tbsp tomato purée
1 tbsp Dijon mustard
white or black pepper
extra-virgin olive oil

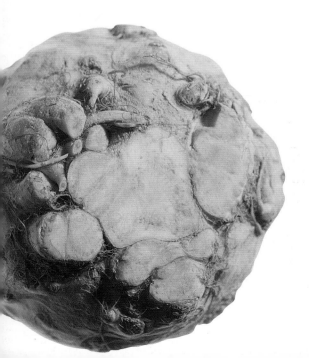

Sweet Potato Fishcakes

Sweet potatoes are a rich source of vitamin C and magnesium, which are both essential in supporting the adrenal glands and thus play an important role in tempering stress. Sweet potato also binds to heavy metals in the gut, so it will help to remove excess toxins. Salmon is a good source of essential fats that support brain function and enhance immune function, while tomatoes contain many antioxidant compounds, in particular lycopene.

Preheat the oven to 400°F/200°C/gas mark 6.

Peel the sweet potatoes, then simmer in boiling water for 15 minutes until tender. Allow to cool, then mash them. Mix together the sweet potato and half the salmon, the tomato purée, mustard and pepper until it is a smooth paste. Add the remaining salmon, then shape into fishcakes and refrigerate for at least 1 hour.

Heat a little olive oil in a frying pan and put the fishcakes in to brown very lightly on each side, then place in the oven for 15 minutes. Do not allow the fishcakes to burn, either in the oil or in the oven.

Serve on a bed of steamed spinach or shredded celeriac (if you have not used the latter in making the fishcakes).

Variations: add dill or coriander to the fishcake mixture.

Roast Cod with Pesto

Cod is a low-fat white fish that contains selenium, calcium and magnesium, thereby supporting the stress response, fighting free radicals and boosting the immune system. Pine nuts contain B vitamins and zinc, and are a good source of protein (B vitamins are used in the process of energy production at cellular level).

4oz/100g basil leaves
4oz/100g pine nuts
4 tbsp olive oil
black pepper
1 piece of cod (4oz/100g) per person

Preheat the oven to 400°F/200°C/gas mark 6.

To make the pesto, combine the basil leaves, pine nuts and olive oil with some freshly ground black pepper in a blender. Blend for a minute or so (if you prefer your pesto more coarse, blend for just 45 seconds).

Roast the cod in the oven for 12 minutes, then remove from the oven. Using a spoon, paste some pesto on the fish. Serve with vegetables.

Variations: add Parmesan cheese to the pesto mixture; replace the basil with tarragon for an interesting flavour alternative.

Middle Eastern Spiced Sea Bass

Like all fish, sea bass is a rich source of essential fats, which support the immune system and can improve cognitive function. Cumin and cardamom seeds have a warming effect on the body.

4 sea-bass fillets
2 tbsp olive oil
2 tsp coriander leaves, chopped
1 tbsp paprika
1 tbsp cumin seeds
5 cardamom seeds
juice of 1 lime
black pepper

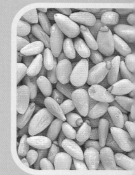

Preheat the oven to 400°F/200°C/gas mark 6.

Place the sea-bass fillets in an ovenproof dish. Combine the olive oil, herbs and spices with the lime juice and some freshly ground black pepper, then pour over the sea bass. Ensure that the fish is well covered and leave to marinate for at least an hour.

Place the covered dish in the oven for 15 minutes, then serve with steamed vegetables.

Variation: if sea bass is not available, try substituting cod or halibut.

Chicken and Chickpea Stew

Chicken is a good source of the B vitamins that are involved in energy production, while chickpeas contain both minerals and protein, and are beneficial to the kidneys and digestive tract.

14oz/400g chickpeas, pre-soaked for 24 hours
1 onion, finely chopped
1 clove of garlic, finely chopped
3 tbsp olive oil
1 tsp paprika
1 tsp dried rosemary
2 chicken breasts
2 chicken legs
14oz/400g tomatoes, chopped

Soak the chickpeas in water overnight, remove any residue from the water's surface, then bring to the boil and simmer for 30 minutes. Drain and leave to cool. Alternatively, canned chickpeas will suffice, as long as they are sugar- and salt-free.

Preheat the oven to 400°F/200°C/gas mark 6.

Sauté the onion and garlic in the olive oil until they are translucent, but do not burn. Stir in the paprika and rosemary, then remove from the heat.

Place the chicken in an ovenproof dish and roast for 20 minutes. Remove from the oven and transfer to a frying pan with the onion and herb mix. Turn the meat a few times so that the chicken is well covered, then stir in the chickpeas and tomatoes. Cover and simmer for 40 minutes.

Variation: replace the chickpeas with any vegetable you like, cut into pieces – broccoli, carrots, parsnips and potatoes work well, to make this a more traditional stew.

Bean and Spinach Soup

Kidney beans are high in fibre, which can help to remove excess cholesterol and toxins from the colon. Spinach is a rich source of minerals, is thought to be anti-cancerous and supports the immune system.

12oz/350g kidney beans
1 tbsp olive oil
3 leeks, sliced
2 cloves of garlic, crushed
3 small potatoes, peeled and cubed
3 bay leaves
6 sprigs of lemon thyme
32fl oz/950ml vegetable stock
1lb 2oz/500g fresh spinach, washed
juice of 2 lemons

Soak the beans in water overnight, then bring to the boil and allow to boil for 30 minutes. Reduce the heat and simmer for 1 hour, removing any residue from the surface of the water (alternatively, buy tinned beans without added sugar or salt).

To a large pan add the oil, leeks and garlic and gently sauté until soft, without letting anything burn. Add the potatoes, bay leaves and lemon thyme, together with the stock and the beans. Simmer for 40 minutes. Serve in warmed bowls, stirring in the spinach and lemon juice just before serving.

Variations: replace the potatoes with one sweet potato; replace the spinach with watercress.

Steamed Whole Fish with Cucumber and Almonds

All fish contains essential fats and minerals, such as calcium, magnesium and selenium. Most fish contains vitamin D as well, making it a good source of nutrients for bone health. Cucumber is a source of antioxidants and can have a mild diuretic effect while aiding digestion. Almonds are rich in minerals, in addition to leatril, which is thought to have an anti-cancer effect.

Serves 2

Mix together the garlic and ginger. Peel the cucumber and slice it lengthways, then mix with the garlic and ginger and place in an ovenproof dish. Place the whole fish on top, then pour the rice wine over the fish.Scatter the shallots on top. Boil some water in a large pan, then place the dish in a steamer over the boiling water. Cover and steam for 12 minutes. Remove the fish, sprinkle the almonds on top and drizzle with sesame oil. Serve the finished dish with soy sauce.

1 large clove of garlic, crushed
2 tbsp grated ginger
1 medium cucumber
1 large whole fresh fish, such as trout
2 tbsp rice wine
1 shallot, cut into strips
4oz/100g flaked almonds
2 tbsp sesame oil
light soy sauce
5oz/150g rice noodles

Meanwhile cook the rice noodles in boiling water for 3 minutes. Drain and run under the hot tap to remove any excess starch. Shake off the water and serve with a little sesame oil as a side-dish.

Variations: use tuna or turbot instead of trout; replace the cucumber with some red chilli, deseeded and cut into strips, for added spice and flavour.

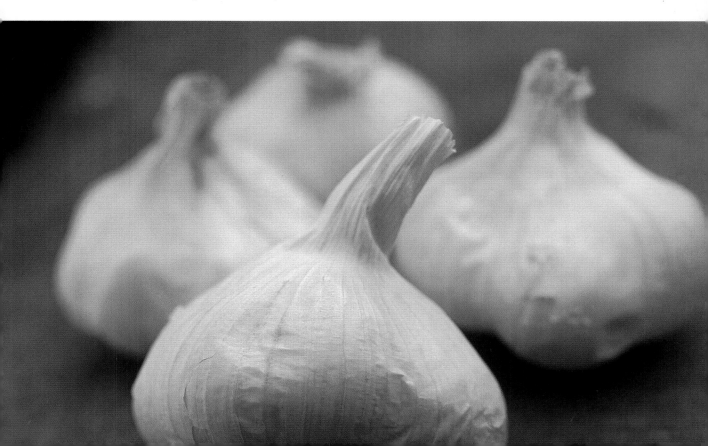

Roast Cumin Chicken and Beets

Cumin has a warming effect on the body. Chicken is a good source of protein and contains vitamin A, B_3 and B_6, plus the minerals potassium and magnesium. The B group of vitamins is essential for energy production. Beetroot is thought to have detoxifying properties.

8 whole beetroots, with the
    stems trimmed
4 chicken breasts
2 tbsp olive oil
2 tsp cumin seeds
1 tbsp balsamic vinegar
2 tbsp dried oregano

Preheat the oven to 350°F/180°C/gas mark 4. Place the beetroots in an ovenproof dish and bake for 40 minutes.

Take the chicken breasts, remove any skin, then drizzle with 1 tbsp of olive oil and a sprinkling of cumin seeds. Remove the beets from the oven, add the chicken and replace in the oven for 15 minutes.

To make the dressing, mix 1 tbsp of olive oil, the balsamic vinegar and the oregano in a small bowl. Drizzle it over the chicken and beets and serve immediately.

Variation: replace the beetroot with parsnips.

Tuna Salad

Tuna contains essential fats and selenium, which is a potent antioxidant. It is also low in fat and a good source of protein. Tomatoes and cucumbers provide further antioxidants, such as lycopene and vitamin C.

Cut the tuna into thick chunks, then marinate it in a bowl with 1 tbsp of the soy sauce and the rice wine. Mix the tomatoes and cucumber with the salad leaves.

To make the dressing, combine 2 tbsp of the soy sauce, the lime juice and sesame oil. Mix well with a fork.

Heat some oil in a frying pan and sear the tuna for 1 minute on each side. Place it amid the salad and serve with the dressing drizzled on top.

12oz/350g fresh tuna
3 tbsp light soy sauce
1 tbsp rice wine
5oz/150g cherry tomatoes
1 cucumber, chopped
11oz/300g salad leaves
1 tbsp lime juice
2 tbsp sesame oil
extra-virgin olive oil for sautéing

Variation: use any fish you want, if tuna is not available – swordfish works well, but should be cooked so that it is slightly underdone when it is removed from the heat; allowing the fish to cool a little will provide enough time for it to cook through in its own heat, without overcooking.

Poached Lemon Chicken with Angel-Hair Pasta

Chicken is a primary protein source as well as being low in fat (once the skin is removed). Lemons contain antioxidant properties, while parsley has beneficial effects on the cardiovascular system.

2 large lemons
4 chicken breasts
1³/₄pt/1l chicken stock
11oz/300g angel-hair pasta (very thin spaghetti)
7oz/200g low-fat crème fraîche
black pepper
4oz/100g flat-leaf parsley, chopped, plus a few leaves for garnish

Bring a large pan of water to the boil, then add the juice of half a lemon. Place the chicken breasts in the simmering water for 10 minutes, then remove and cut the meat into cubes.

Meanwhile, in another pan, bring 1 litre of chicken stock to the boil. Cook the pasta in the stock for 5 minutes, then drain.

In a small pan, warm the juice from the remaining lemons with the crème fraîche, freshly ground black pepper and chopped parsley.

Replace the pasta in a pan, adding the crème fraîche and lemon mixture together with the cubes of chicken. Warm for 2 minutes over a medium heat and serve, garnished with a few parsley leaves.

Variation: veal works well instead of chicken – grill the veal slices (one per person) and allow to cook (the veal should be slightly underdone); cut into strips and add to the sauce, combining well to mix the flavours.

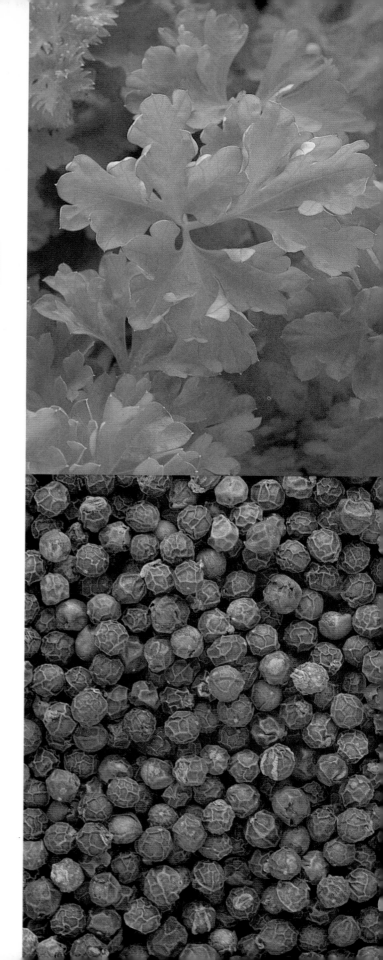

Braised Tofu with Tomatoes and Aubergines

Tofu is a vegetarian source of protein and is renowned for helping to balance hormone levels. It is also thought to be anti-cancerous and, coupled with the lycopene and beta-carotene contained in the tomato and aubergine respectively, makes this dish an excellent source of a wide range of anti-cancer substances.

extra-virgin olive oil for frying

14oz/400g tofu, cubed

1 tbsp rice wine

1 large onion, chopped

1 can chopped tomatoes (without added sugar or salt)

11oz/300g aubergine, sliced lengthways

Warm some olive oil in a frying pan, add the tofu and sauté very gently until a little browning occurs (usually in about 8 minutes). Remove from the heat, sprinkle with the rice wine and set aside.

Sauté the onion in some more olive oil until it is translucent, then add the tomatoes and aubergines and cook over a gentle heat until the vegetables have broken down a bit. Add the tofu pieces, warm through and serve.

Variation: replace the aubergine with peppers (one per person), using different-coloured peppers to make this dish even more attractive.

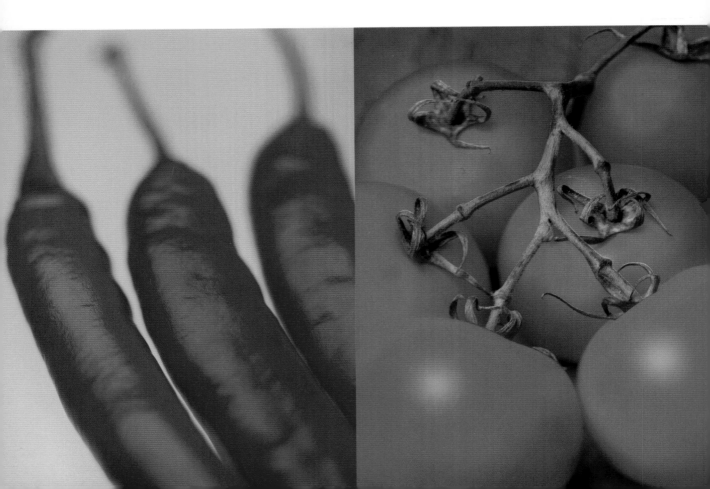

Asian Fish Broth with Salmon

Ginger is thought to improve the circulation and prevent nausea. Salmon is a rich source of immune-supporting and stress-regulating minerals, as well as essential fats.

Warm the fish stock (preferably use fresh fish stock, which is available from most supermarkets) in a large saucepan, adding the lime leaves, lemongrass, ginger, chilli peppers and some freshly ground white pepper. Bring to the boil, then reduce the heat and simmer for 25 minutes, allowing the flavours to infuse.

1³/₄pt/1l fresh fish stock
3 lime leaves
2 stalks of lemongrass
1 large piece of peeled fresh ginger
2 red chilli peppers, deseeded and sliced
white pepper
7oz/200g skinless salmon fillet
2oz/50g coriander leaves

Using a sharp knife, cut the salmon into strips and add it to the broth. Leave the pan on the lowest heat for 8 minutes, then add the coriander leaves and serve immediately.

Variations: to make a heartier broth, add some rice noodles, or some sliced vegetables such as cucumber and broccoli, to the liquid for 3 minutes before serving; replace the salmon with any white fish of your choice.

Pasta with Prawns, Lime and Lemon

Prawns are a source of selenium and zinc, both of which support the immune system. Zinc is also essential for repair and healing. Pasta is a complex carbohydrate that easily converts to glucose in the body. Lemons and limes are both good sources of antioxidants and are believed to have anti-cancer properties, as does broccoli, which also stimulates liver action.

1lb 2oz/500g large raw, peeled prawns
1 tbsp olive oil
2 tsp black pepper
1 tsp ground coriander
1lb 2oz/500g pasta (any shape and flavour: chilli pasta works well)
9oz/250g broccoli florets, cut into small pieces
oil for frying
4 heads of pak choi
2oz/50g basil leaves
juice of 1 lemon and 1 lime

Combine the prawns with the olive oil, pepper and coriander. Boil a large saucepan of water, add the pasta and cook until al dente. Remove from the heat and drain. Steam the broccoli over boiling water until it, too, is al dente.

Heat the prawns in a hot frying pan with a little oil for 1 minute on each side, then toss them into the pasta, adding the broccoli, pak choi and basil. Pour on the lemon and lime juice and serve immediately.

Variations: instead of prawns, try adding fresh scallops (sautéed in a little olive oil on a low heat for 6 minutes, then added to the cooked pasta, covered and allowed to for 5 minutes before serving); if you prefer to avoid shellfish, then cooked chicken cut into strips works well with this sauce.

vegetable and grain recipes

These recipes for grains and vegetables all make excellent side-dishes to any of the main courses featured on pp. 112–19. You could also try one as a light lunch or make some extra as a snack. However, do remember that they lack protein, although they do contain fibre, so they are best used as accompaniments to a main dish.

All recipes serve four people.

Mushroom and Pak Choi Stir-Fry

Mushrooms contain B vitamins and minerals, and are thought to be beneficial for thinning the blood and supporting immune function. Pak choi contains fibre and antioxidant nutrients, while garlic is believed to be antiviral and antibiotic.

4 heads of pak choi

4oz/100g shiitake mushrooms

4oz/100g button mushrooms

2 tbsp peanut oil

2 cloves of garlic, crushed

1 tbsp cold water

4 spring onions, chopped and
    with the ends removed

1 tbsp soy sauce

1 tbsp rice wine

Wash all the vegetables thoroughly, then pat dry on kitchen paper.

Heat the oil in a wok. Add the garlic and pak choi, and stir-fry for 1 minute. Add the cold water and mushrooms, and stir-fry for another minute. Add the spring onions, soy sauce and rice wine and stir for 1 minute. Serve at once.

Variation: try adding bean sprouts and shredded courgettes for a different flavour.

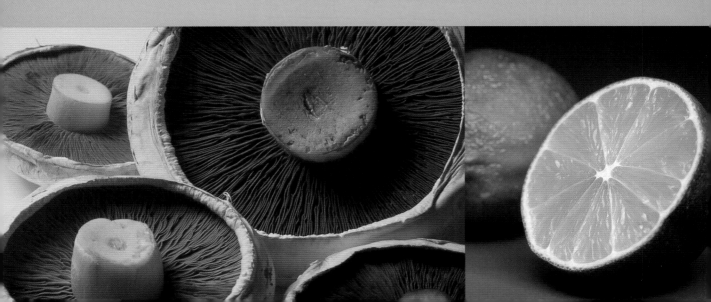

Thai Lime Rice

Brown rice contains many of the B vitamins and is rich in minerals. It is also thought to be calming to the nervous system. Brown rice should be used in favour of white rice, many varieties of which have been 'polished' to achieve their colouring and have lost nutrients in the process.

1lb 6oz/600g brown rice
3 cups water
2 tbsp Thai fish sauce
2 stalks of lemongrass, finely sliced
4 lime leaves
grated zest of 2 limes
2 tbsp lime juice

Wash the rice several times in cool water, then place all the ingredients in a saucepan and bring to the boil. As soon as the liquid is boiling, cover and reduce the heat to low, then cook for 25 minutes. Remove from the heat, leave to stand for 5 minutes without removing the cover, and then serve.

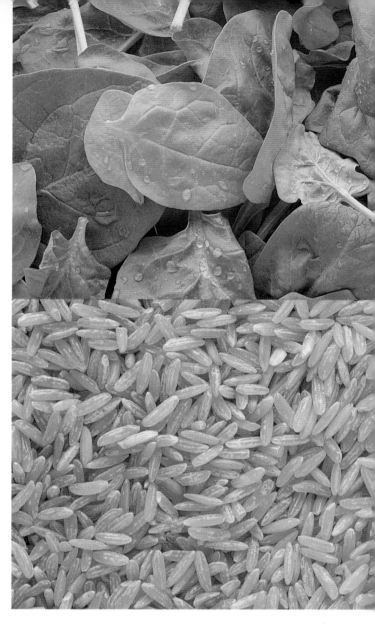

Spinach with Spring Onions

Spinach contains antioxidant nutrients and is a perfect anti-cancer food. Onions are beneficial to the cardio-vascular system, while olive oil is a rich source of mono-unsaturated fats, which are beneficial to the heart and immune system.

1 large bunch of spring onions
3 tbsp extra-virgin olive oil
1lb/450g fresh, washed spinach
$1/4$ nutmeg, freshly grated
black pepper

Chop the spring onions, discarding the rough ends, and add them to a saucepan with the oil. Warm over a low to medium heat until they have softened a little (usually about 5 minutes). Do not allow the oil to burn. Add the spinach and combine it with the oil and spring onions, stirring until the leaves have reduced (usually within 1 minute).

Serve in a warm dish, or on individual plates, sprinkled with the nutmeg and freshly ground black pepper.

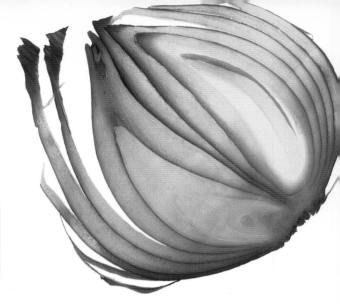

Baby Potato Salad

Potatoes are high in vitamin C, yet boiling them may reduce their overall content. Balance this by serving this salad as a side-dish to another vegetable.

1lb 12oz/800g baby or new
    potatoes, washed
1 large red onion, chopped
7oz/200g low-fat crème fraîche

City Dressing

$3^1/_2$fl oz/100ml extra-virgin olive oil
1fl oz/25ml white-wine vinegar
1 level tsp English mustard powder
zest and juice of 1 unwaxed lemon, or
    lime if you prefer
freshly ground black pepper to taste

Combine all the ingredients in a clean, dry bottle, seal tightly and shake well.

In a saucepan, boil the potatoes for 20 minutes. Remove from the heat and drain, then allow to cool for a while. When the potatoes are cool enough to work with, cut them into cubes (or any shape you like) and add them to a bowl.

Add the onion to the dressing, then cover the potatoes well with it. Just before serving, add the crème fraîche, and combine so that all the ingredients are well mixed.

Variation: add 2oz/50g chopped flat-leaf parsley or basil to the potato salad.

City Tabbouleh

Bulgar wheat is high in B vitamins and minerals, so it provides energy and supports the immune function. Tomatoes are the primary source of lycopene, a potent antioxidant, while parsley cleanses the blood and helps create a more alkaline environment.

5fl oz/150ml vegetable stock
7oz/200g bulgar wheat
2 cans chopped tomatoes (without
    added sugar or salt)
4oz/100g flat-leaf parsley
4oz/100g coriander or mint leaves

Warm the vegetable stock in a large saucepan, then add the bulgar wheat and bring to the boil. Turn down the heat to the lowest setting. Cover and allow to simmer gently for 20 minutes, until the wheat has absorbed all the stock.

Allow to cool, then stir in the tomatoes, parsley and the coriander or mint leaves and serve.

Classic Risotto

Like soup, risotto can be an extremely versatile dish and is easy to make, as long as you are prepared to stand and stir continuously while it is cooking. Remember that you will need to balance this high-carbohydrate dish with some protein and fibre.

Risotto rice contains B vitamins and minerals, yet the main source of antioxidants will come from whatever vegetable you add or serve at the same meal.

Warm the stock so that it is just bubbling.

Meanwhile, dice the onion and heat it in the oil in a deep saucepan with high sides (it is worth investing in a risotto pan if you do not have a suitable saucepan). Stir the onion, allowing it to become translucent, but do not let the oil burn or the onion brown.

At this stage you can add the vegetables that you intend to use, such as mushrooms, broccoli or asparagus – in fact, anything you like (suggestions follow this recipe).

> 2^1/$_2$pt/1.5l vegetable or chicken stock
> 1 large onion
> 3 tbsp extra-virgin olive oil
> approx. 7oz/200g fresh vegetables of your
>   choice, chopped (see below)
> 11oz/300g arborio rice
> 1 glass of dry white wine (optional)

Now add the rice and fold it into the onion mixture, ensuring that all the rice is coated with oil. Add the wine, if desired, and allow the rice to absorb the liquid, stirring it gently all the time. Then, ladle by ladle, add the bubbling stock, stirring it in and allowing the rice to absorb all the liquid before you add the next ladle. (If you are adding a herb, you can do so at any time.) Keep stirring until all the stock has been used, which should take approximately 20 minutes. Serve the risotto immediately in warm soup bowls.

SUGGESTED ADDITIONS

Mushrooms – work well with parsley or green peppercorns

Broad beans – combines well with fresh mint

Asparagus – keep some steamed asparagus back to add when the dish is cooked

Broccoli – retain some small florets to garnish the finished dish

Chicken – poach the chicken, or add plain, grilled chicken slices at the very end

Pumpkin – add early on in the cooking process

Squash – add towards the end of cooking to retain the colour

Salmon – add cooked salmon at the very end, and use fish stock in place of the chicken or vegetable stock

Cod – again use fish stock

Prawns – add 5 minutes before the rice is finished, and allow to cook; keep back one cooked prawn per person to place on top on the risotto when you serve it.

smoothies

Smoothies make a perfect breakfast or snack. They are an excellent combination of protein and carbohydrates. As fresh fruit is used in every smoothie, they are naturally high in the antioxidants that are so essential to combat free radicals.

All recipes serve four people.

Classic City Smoothie

The basic smoothie recipe is very easy to make and can be adapted to taste. If you prefer a smoother texture, then use slightly less tofu; if you prefer a thicker smoothie, add a little extra!

14oz/400g plain tofu (preferably organic), cut into cubes
$2^1/_4$pt/1.25l soya, rice or oat milk (unsweetened)
fruit of your choice (see below for suggestions)
1 lump of ice (optional)

Place all the ingredients in a blender, then blend until the mixture is free of either fruit or tofu lumps. If you are not used to eating tofu, then use smaller quantities at first.

Banana Berry Smoothie

The banana gives this combination a lovely smooth texture and contains pectin, which is useful for removing toxins and heavy metals from the digestive tract. The berries are high in beta-carotene and vitamin C and have anti-cancer properties.

2 bananas
11oz/300g mixed berries, such as blackberries, strawberries and blueberries

Pear and Peach Smoothie

Pears give this smoothie a grainy texture and, like bananas, they contain pectin. Peaches contain minerals and antioxidants and are easily digestible.

2 pears, deseeded and cut into quarters
2 peaches, with the stones removed, cut into quarters

Prune and Kiwi Smoothie

The prunes do not completely blend in, giving an interesting texture and an intense flavour. They are useful for the cardiovascular system, as they reduce cholesterol, while kiwi fruit are a rich source of vitamin C and minerals (which are found in the seeds).

8 prunes, pitted
3 kiwi fruit, peeled

Orange and Apricot Smoothie

This combination delivers a high degree of antioxidants, and as apricots contain boron, which is essential for healthy bones, it can be useful for building bone strength.

2 large oranges, peeled and quartered
6 fresh apricots, pitted and halved

Apple and Frozen Strawberry Smoothie

This is a delicious ice-cold treat that is perfect for a hot day – children also love this one, as it resembles ice cream or frozen yoghurt. Apples are a rich source of pectin, which removes toxins from the bowels. Strawberries are high in antioxidant vitamins and are thought to be antiviral and anti-cancerous as well.

7oz/200g fresh strawberries, frozen for at least 3 hours
3 large apples, deseeded and quartered

Smoothie tips

Vary the content of your smoothies, so that you benefit from a wide variety of fruits.

For the taste of chocolate without the sugar, add a teaspoon of organic cocoa powder (not drinking-chocolate powder).

Add a tablespoon of live, unsweetened yoghurt for variety.

Add some fresh seeds, such as pumpkin or sesame, to the mixture before you blend it, ensuring that the seeds are properly ground before you drink the smoothie. In this way you can benefit from the essential fats and minerals that seeds contain.

Add a tablespoon of sugar-free frozen yoghurt to create a frozen shake texture.

Do not use dried fruits – they are high in sugar and can have mould on their surface that is invisible to the eye.

five fast lunches

You do not have to cook something complicated to get all the benefits that food can offer. Here are five examples of quick, light lunches that will deliver complex carbohydrates, first-class protein, vegetable fibre and abundant flavour. Each dish should be served with a salad comprising salad leaves and at least two vegetables – preferably raw (perhaps grated or chopped carrot, courgette, broccoli or watercress) – accompanied by City Dressing (see p. 122) if desired.

Each recipe serves one person.

Any of the main courses (see pp. 112–119) would also be excellent for lunch if you have a little more time in which to make them.

Poached Eggs with Rice Salad

Grate the vegetables into a bowl, then add the salad leaves and brown rice and mix well.

Poach the eggs lightly in boiling water, then place them on the rice and vegetables and top with City Dressing (see p. 122).

> 1 large carrot
> 1 sweet potato
> 3oz/75g salad leaves
> 1 cup cooked brown rice
> 2 large eggs

Mushroom Omelette

Break the eggs into a small bowl and mix vigorously with a fork.

In a small non-stick pan, heat a knob of butter over a medium heat. Add the mushrooms and let them sauté gently for 4 minutes, stirring them frequently with a wooden spoon. Remove the mushrooms and set aside.

> 2 large eggs
> knob of butter
> 7oz/200g mushrooms, washed and
>   chopped
> black pepper
> 3oz/75g salad leaves

Pour the egg mixture into the pan, which should still have a layer of melted butter in it. With the heat still at medium, cover the pan with a lid and leave on the heat for 3 minutes. Then remove the cover, and place the cooked mushrooms on one side of the flat omelette. Grind some black pepper on top. Now carefully put a fish slice under the opposite side of the omelette and fold it over, so that it covers the mushrooms. Cover again with the lid for 1 minute, then serve on a bed of salad leaves, being careful that you do not lose too many mushrooms.

Baked Potato with Bean Salad

Preheat the oven to 400°F/200°C/gas mark 6.

Wash the potato and pierce it at least five times with a sharp knife. Place in the hot oven for at least 1 hour 10 minutes, but do not let the skin burn, merely brown.

1 large baking potato
1 x 1lb/450g can of mixed beans (in water, without added sugar and salt)
1 small red onion
1 tsp olive or walnut oil

Meanwhile, wash the beans thoroughly under the cold tap and pat dry on a cloth. Chop the onion and mix it with the beans. Top with City Dressing (see p. 122).

When the potato is cooked, remove it from the oven and cut it in half. Drizzle the oil over the potato flesh, then mix it in with a fork. Serve it with the bean salad.

Sardines with Herbed Rye Toast

Mix the dill with the olive oil, then spread on the rye bread, cover with the sliced tomato and place under a hot grill for 2 minutes.

1 bunch of dill, finely chopped
1 tsp olive oil
2 slices rye bread
1 large tomato, sliced
1 can sardines
black pepper

Drain the sardines of the oil, then place them on top of the tomatoes, sprinkle with freshly ground black pepper and serve.

Basilled Chicken

Warm the chicken stock and half the basil leaves in a saucepan over a medium high heat, bringing it to a slow boil. Place the chicken in the pan and cover, then leave to cook for 10 minutes. Remove the chicken and basil leaves from the pan and place them on a plate.

$1^3/_4$pt/1l vegetable stock (see p. 107)
3oz/75g fresh basil leaves
1 fresh chicken breast (without skin)

When the chicken has cooled a little, slice it into strips and add to your chosen vegetable salad along with the wilted basil leaves. Top with City Dressing (see p. 122), garnish with the remainder of the basil leaves and serve.

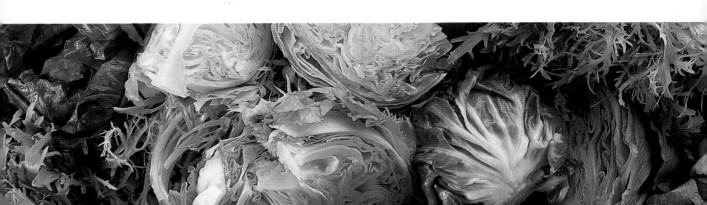

eating out

Restaurants are an integral part of city living, so much so that many people seem to eat out as often as they eat at home. Eating out does not, however, mean that you cannot eat optimally, although some cuisines offer more versatility than others.

Bear in mind that ideally you need to eat some protein, in the form of tofu, fish, poultry, eggs, meat or beans. Carbohydrates should be unrefined and complex – wholewheat bread or pasta, brown rice or any grain. Vegetables should make up a large proportion of your meal. You could start with a selection of leaves and a little tuna or chicken; or a totally vegetable-based dish. Follow with the protein of your choice (grilled, roast, baked or poached), plenty of crisp vegetables and some carbohydrates in the form of a few new potatoes, a little pasta or some rice.

There is one problem: how best to finish your meal. Traditionally we like to have something sweet. Fruit is not advisable after a protein meal, as it contains enzymes that can speed up the digestion of the protein, potentially encouraging undigested foods to enter the colon. Instead, choose the lightest dish that you can – perhaps get one to share. But good health can afford some lapses, so if you have been eating well, then having a chocolate dessert once in while is unlikely to cause any ill-effects.

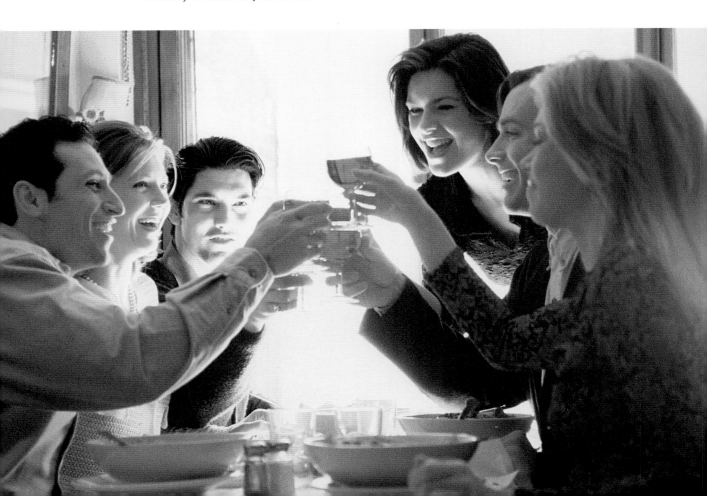

Here are some basic guidelines to help you achieve the best balance from different cuisines.

French

French food can easily work well for you, but you need to ensure that what you order is not overly rich in fats, which are often hidden in sauces. If you choose a classic French onion soup, do not have all the cheese and avoid the croûtons, as they may be high in fats. Main courses in French restaurants are easy to select, and combining food groups can be achieved without too much effort.

Indian

Indian food tends to be high in fats and carbohydrates, but if you avoid the creamy sauces and large quantities of rice and bread, then you will be more likely not to feel excessively full after you have eaten. Choose a vegetable-based dish to start, and share some naan bread. Tandoori chicken is a good alternative to a dish with sauce, but do ask if food colourings have been used to create the colour on the chicken, instead of the traditional Tandoori methods, which take longer to achieve. Vegetables are plentiful in Indian restaurants, so order more than one dish and favour those that are not cooked in excess oil or ghee.

Italian

Italian food (in addition to Asian) is perhaps the cuisine best suited to optimal eating. Many appetizers are vegetable-based; and although pasta is a good source of complex carbohydrates, it is perhaps advisable to have some as a starter instead of a larger portion for your main course, when you risk not getting any protein with your meal. For the main course you might select chicken, fish or even occasionally some red meat, simply grilled and served with a selection of fresh vegetables. Like pasta, risotto is very high in carbohydrates and should be eaten at lunch instead of dinner, to give you a greater chance to use up the energy that the rice will provide.

Chinese

Chinese food is often light and offers an excellent opportunity to eat crisp vegetables alongside good protein sources. Stir-fried food is not ideal, however, as the fats used are sensitive to heat, although as the food is not overcooked the potential damage is limited. Once again, do not eat too much rice, but let the bulk of your meal come from vegetables and protein, with some carbohydrates making up the remainder.

Japanese

Japanese food is an ideal way to eat in the city. Sushi is readily available and does not have to be expensive, although many commercially available varieties add sugar to the rice. Miso soup, seaweed and tempura are all light, easily digestible and have many positive qualities. Again, do not fill up on the white rice that comes with the sushi or as a side-dish, but add some sashimi to provide essential fats.

energy day

Whether you need extra energy because you have a long day ahead or an important event such as an exam or a presentation, maximizing energy is a vital part of city life. You can follow this one-day plan either the day before the event and on the day itself, or just on the day in question, although the latter will not have quite the same beneficial results.

The usual guidelines apply: avoid all high-sugar foods and drinks that provide short-term energy. A more consistent energy is preferable to highs and lows. The emphasis of this programme is on protein and complex carbohydrates, with added vegetables and fruit.

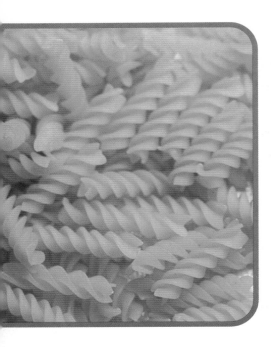

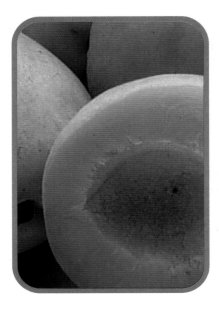

Supplements

Nutritional supplements may help maximize your energy. For physical energy consider the following supplements, all of which are involved in the process of creating energy at cellular level. The recommended daily levels are general guidelines only; since each individual's requirements differ, according to age, personal situation and health status, you may like to seek the advice of a qualified nutritional consultant concerning your own biochemical status. Supplements are best taken in the morning with food, perhaps immediately after breakfast:

> **B-complex: high-strength tablet containing the whole range of B vitamins**
> **Co-enzyme Q10 (also known as CoQ10): 50mg**
> **Chromium: 400mcg**
> **Magnesium: 600mg**
> **Manganese: 15mg**
> **Copper: 1.5mg**
> **Iron: 25mg**

(The last five are best found in a good-quality multivitamin.)

For mental energy the following nutrients would be appropriate:

> **Choline: 50mg**
> **Magnesium taurate: 200mg (100mg twice daily, not with food)**
> **Ginkgo biloba: 450mg (150mg three times daily)**
> **B-complex: high-strength tablet**
> **Iron: 25mg**
> **Chromium: 400mcg**

Breakfast

One piece of fruit, such as an apple, pear or banana

Two scrambled eggs or a two-egg omelette with
one slice of rye or wheat-free bread or sugar-
free muesli with fresh fruit (not dried), plain
yoghurt and soya milk

Caffeine-free tea, such as peppermint or green tea,
or one cup of decaffeinated coffee (ensuring that
is has been processed using the water method)

Mid-morning snack

Two pieces of fresh fruit, such as kiwi fruit, orange,
mango, cherries or apricots

A palmful of mixed pumpkin, sesame and
sunflower seeds or two oat cakes with sesame
spread (tahini) or fish pâté

Lunch

Any vegetable soup (see pp. 106–107)

Grilled, steamed or stir-fried chicken or fish

Three portions of vegetables, cooked yet crisp

One small serving of brown rice or wholewheat pasta

Mid-afternoon snack

Raw vegetables or fruit

Sugar-free nut butter on rice or oat cakes

Dinner

Choose a different protein from the type you had at
lunch, but ensure that you have poultry, fish, tofu
or eggs (if you did not have eggs for breakfast)

Two portions of fresh vegetables

A few strands of pasta or a little brown rice or lentils

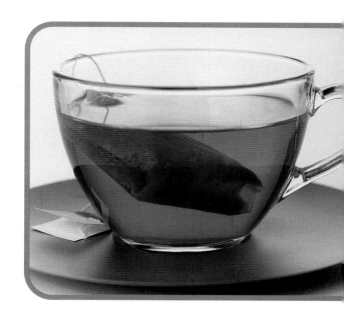

Essential oils

You could also improve your alertness by burning some essential oils, or adding some to your
bath (do not apply them directly to the skin, as they must be combined with a base oil such as
almond oil). Rosemary and peppermint oil are both stimulating (as such they should not be
used at night), while basil oil helps you focus and clear the mind; lemongrass oil helps to
counter physical fatigue.

calming day

If you want to follow a programme that is more calming and will help you rest and relax, then the following plan should benefit you. Ensure that you drink plenty of water throughout the day, and avoid sugar and caffeine. The emphasis of this programme is on vegetables and fruit, as opposed to protein and complex carbohydrates.

Breakfast

Classic City Smoothie (see p. 124)
Two pieces of fruit with plain yoghurt and a
    teaspoon of linseeds
Ginger or peppermint tea
Oat porridge with soya milk and fruit

Mid-morning snack

One piece of fruit
A palmful of raw almonds or cashews

Lunch

Onion or parsnip soup
Salad comprising a variety of lettuce leaves, raw
    broccoli, raw sweet potato (shredded) and any
two other vegetables of your choice, plus tofu
    or fish
City Dressing (see p. 122)

Mid-afternoon snack

Two pieces of fruit
Camomile or ginger tea

Dinner

Miso or vegetable soup
Grilled fish or chicken, or braised tofu
Three portions of steamed vegetables

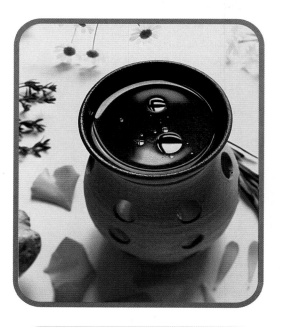

Supplements

Some supplements are thought to
    relax the body, in particular:
Magnesium: 600mg
Vitamin B$_5$: 500mg
Vitamin B$_3$: 100mg
**Vitamin C: 3000mg (1000mg three
    times daily).**

Essential oils

You could enhance this programme by investing in some calming essential oils to add to your bath or burn in a vaporizer, such as geranium, lavender, mandarin or frankincense. Or put a drop of essential oil on your pillow, handkerchief or jacket collar. Never place essential oils directly onto the skin, but combine with a base oil, such as almond oil, instead.

weekend detoxification plan

As we have seen, many health issues can be exacerbated by living in the city. Undertaking a detoxification process can help your overall health by allowing some of the stored toxins that have built up over time to be released.

During this period you may experience any number of symptoms, ranging from a dry mouth, headaches, fatigue and muscle ache to irritability and a reduction in cognitive function. Your skin may show signs of stress, as the skin is used as an elimination route for the toxins. So do not be surprised if you develop minor spots or a light rash for the duration of the weekend.

Choose your weekend well in advance, ensuring that it is one you can leave free of arrangements and commitments. You will need to rest and sleep, so staying at home as much as possible is advisable.

Preparing for your weekend

It is not advisable to jump straight into a detoxification programme. A few days' preparation can improve the efficiency of the removal of toxins. Ideally you should be able to be at home by late afternoon on Friday, ready to begin.

The previous Monday you should increase the amount of fruits and vegetables that you eat by at least two pieces. Increase this again on Tuesday and Wednesday, so that by the Thursday you are eating at least six pieces of fruit and having six different servings of vegetables.

At the same time your alcohol consumption should be reduced to zero by Wednesday, and protein from animal sources should be reduced gradually throughout the week, so that by Thursday evening you have finished whatever protein you have in stock at home (aside from tofu and beans).

Aim to be drinking at least $3^1/_2$pt/2l of water daily by Thursday, cutting out all teas and coffees (even herbal and decaffeinated) by Thursday evening.

Shopping list

You need to ensure that you have the following items at home:

1 carton of vegetable stock or $3^1/_2$pt/2l fresh home-made vegetable stock

vegetable bouillon powder (available from health-food stores)

10 green apples

9 x $1^3/_4$pt/1l bottles of still mineral water

1lb/450g of any white fish, such as cod or haddock

8oz/225g tuna, salmon or mackerel

2 large heads of broccoli

2 heads of green cabbage

20 carrots

2lb/1kg fresh spinach, washed

2lb/1kg fresh beetroot, peeled

1 large piece of fresh ginger

15 nettle leaves, washed (available from Asian supermarkets, health-food stores and greengrocers)

2 large lemons

salad leaves

extra-virgin olive oil

a juicer

Friday

If Friday is a work day for you, or you have commitments, then do try to be home as early as you can.

Begin the detoxification programme by eating a green salad with steamed broccoli added to it – steam the vegetables, then run them under the cold tap so that they remain crisp and colourful. Have only one tablespoon of olive oil on the salad. Accompany this with a bowl or mug of warm vegetable bouillon.

Go to bed early and aim to get up early on Saturday, perhaps by 8 a.m.

Saturday

For breakfast drink some hot water with one slice of lemon and one of ginger. Follow this with a juice made from liquidized carrots, beetroot, spinach and nettle leaves.

Get outside and take a brisk walk in the fresh air, then return home and do at least 15 minutes of gentle stretching exercises, ensuring that you move gently and slowly.

The remainder of the morning should be spent resting and relaxing – without the aid of computers, radios or telephones! Perhaps you could read, or watch an old movie. Avoid entertaining, as you may well be feeling a little tired. If you like, you can have another glass of juice halfway through the morning.

For lunch, have a bowl of warm bouillon. Poach about 1oz/25g of flaked white fish in bouillon for about 5 minutes, and then add brocolli florets, poaching for another five minutes until the brocolli has softened slightly. Serve in a warm soup bowl, eating slowly and chewing well.

After lunch, rest again. During the afternoon drink two more glasses of vegetable juice. Throughout the day you should be drinking at least $4^1/_2$pt/2.5l of water.

For supper, which you should aim to eat early (perhaps around 7 p.m.), have two more bowls of bouillon. Then head off to bed and get to sleep as early as you can.

Sunday

Today should be spent resting, but if you can arrange to have a massage, then the whole process of detoxification will be even more efficient. You should be having only liquid today – no solid food at all.

For breakfast drink some hot water and lemon, and throughout the morning drink more hot water with some sliced fresh ginger (press the ginger in the cup with a spoon or fork to release the ginger essence). You may be experiencing some hunger, which can be addressed by drinking another vegetable juice made from liquidized carrots, cabbage and broccoli, and some warm bouillon whenever you feel pangs, but do not overeat. Drink at least $4^1/_2$pt/2.5l of water during the day.

Stay quiet and warm, and get to sleep as early as possible in the evening.

Monday

Start the week by eating three pieces of whole fruit, such as apples, then ease yourself into the day as smoothly as possible. Snack on fruit all morning. Lunch should consist of green salad leaves with raw vegetables and a small portion of tuna, salmon or mackerel. If you prefer not to eat fish, then have some chicken breast with the skin removed, or if you are vegetarian then tofu is ideal.

After Monday you can gradually resume your normal eating habits. You may find that your appetite is slightly decreased, and many people report that they crave vegetables and fruit afterwards, which is an excellent sign. Even if you do not crave fresh produce, eat a little more than usual to gain maximum benefit from the whole programme. Continue to drink plenty of still mineral water – at least 3$\frac{1}{2}$pt/2l per day.

By Tuesday you should be feeling the benefits of your weekend – you may feel lighter, more energetic and generally better overall.

Detoxification tips

As you have had three days without tea and coffee, why not continue to leave them out of your diet.

If you experience a dry mouth, mild headaches or muscle ache, this is a quite normal side-effect of the detoxification programme.

Fatigue and irritability are also common side-effects.

If you feel unwell at any time, stop the process by eating some cooked brown rice or a baked potato – complex carbohydrates that will gently raise your blood-glucose levels.

Ensure that you drink at least 4$\frac{1}{2}$pt/2.5l of water daily throughout the programme, keeping a bottle of water near you at all times. Do not worry if you find that you urinate more than usual – this is quite normal and is to be expected.

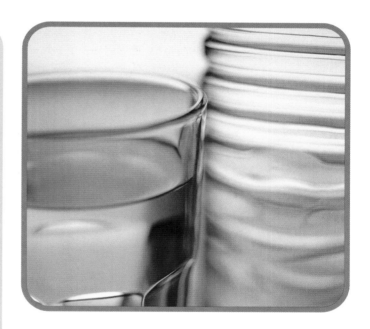

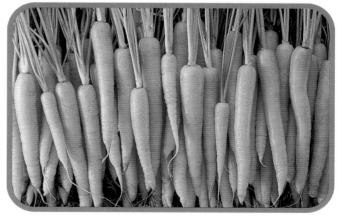

monday-to-friday
weight-management plan

This weight-management plan covers a working week, and should help you lose some body fat, not fluid. So although you may weigh the same at the end, your clothes should be looser and you should feel better in general.

Ensure that you do not have any social commitments for the week, and arrange to exercise at least three times during it, as well as walking more than you would normally do. You will have to put some effort into this programme (and it is not guaranteed to work for everyone), but the investment should be worthwhile.

If you have any existing medical conditions, check with your health professional before undertaking the diet. It is important that you do not follow this plan for longer than one week. It entails reducing your carbohydrate intake, and long-term use could cause serious health conditions, from osteoporosis to muscle loss – none of which is worth risking for a little weight loss.

This five-day plan should have made you more aware of what and how you eat, so take note of this in the ensuing days. The key is to avoid sugar and stimulants, and doing this should help maintain your weight loss. Cook fresh foods whenever possible, and avoid having too many carbohydrates in the evenings, so that they do not get laid down as body fat.

Supplements

Some nutrient supplements are reported to help fat cells release their fat. These do not work for everyone, but may be of help on a programme such as this. It is recommended that you supplement the mineral chromium to a level of 400mcg twice daily (preferably half with breakfast and half with lunch). Chromium is often found to be deficient and assists in facilitating the efficient entry of blood sugar into the cells where it is required.

NB If you have diabetes, you must check with your health practitioner before undertaking any supplementation of chromium.

Basic guidelines

Try to start each day with some exercise, preferably aerobic (see pp. 70–75). You must exercise at least three times during the week.

Drink at least $3^{1}/_{2}$pt/2l of still, bottled mineral water every day.

Choose from any of the suggested breakfasts, snacks, lunches and dinners. Ensure that you do not have the same protein source twice in one day (if you have eggs for breakfast, choose chicken for lunch and fish for dinner).

You should not eat any carbohydrates at all, apart from vegetables, after 4 p.m.

Aim to eat food made at home, and not to rely on shop-bought food.

Eat small, frequent meals – do not skip any meal or snack, even if you do not feel hungry.

Do not overeat.

Breakfast

Alternate the following suggestions – do not have the same thing every day:

Two pieces of fruit, and oat porridge made with water and sprinkled with one teaspoon
  of linseeds

Classic City Smoothie (see p. 124)

Scrambled or poached eggs on rye toast

Fruit salad (made with any three fruits, but preferably one soft and two more fibrous, harder
  fruit, such as a banana, apple and pear) topped with a little plain, low-fat, bio unsweetened
  yoghurt; sprinkle a tablespoon of sesame seeds on top

To drink: green tea, hot water with lemon or ginger slices, peppermint tea, camomile or any
  other herbal tea

Mid-morning or mid-afternoon snack

Choose one of the following:

Two organic oat or rice cakes with cottage cheese

A palmful of mixed pumpkin and sesame seeds

A slice of rye toast or bread with sugar- and salt-free nut butter

Classic City Smoothie (as long as you have not had one for breakfast)

Two pieces of fruit and six raw cashew nuts

Lunch

A large salad made with lettuce and raw spinach leaves, at least three different types of raw
  vegetable, a protein source (chicken, turkey, tuna, salmon, mackerel, tofu or eggs, as long
  as you did not have them for breakfast) and a little cold pasta or brown rice

For variety, add some cooked red or green lentils or a few cooked kidney beans

You may have a slice of rye bread if you have not included the rice or pasta – having both will
  provide excess carbohydrates. Top with City Dressing (see p. 122)

Dinner

Home-made vegetable soup (see pp. 106–107)

One large portion of a protein source, such as grilled chicken, tuna, salmon, cod, haddock,
  sole, carp, sea bass, trout or monkfish

Three types of steamed vegetables

You may use any herbs, such as dill, tarragon, basil or oregano, to add flavour to your meal. Do
  not, however, use any salt – only freshly ground black pepper, if required

NB You must not have carbohydrates in the evenings, except for raw or steamed vegetables.

Late-night snack

If you feel particularly hungry, choose one of the following:

A very small palmful of mixed seeds

six raw almonds or cashews

Once the working week is over, do not rush back into your usual eating habits overnight. The
weekend could all too easily undo your work, if you are not careful.

troubleshooting

Main courses	I am a vegetarian yet many of the suggestions in the book rely on animal products	An excellent source of vegetable protein is tofu, so find as many tofu recipes as you can and learn more about how to use this very versatile food. Beans are also a source of protein, as are nuts and seeds.
Main courses	I prefer meat to fish	Red meat should ideally be limited as it contains saturated fats which encourage imbalances of bacteria in the gut. Poultry is a good compromise, but do try to have some fish, at least three times a week ideally, as it is high in essential fats that protect the heart and promote increased metabolic rate.
Soups	I have a small fridge and cannot store much in it	You could easily make smaller quantities of soup and freeze portions in smaller freeezerproof food containers. This way you will have good nutritious soup on hand for those times when you really do not have time to cook.
General	Garlic - can I leave it out?	If you do not like any one ingredient then feel free to replace it or remove it altogether.
General	Why is there no salt mentioned in any of the recipes?	Salt is not needed to enhance the recipes - each one has its own flavour which will not be helped by the addition of salt. If you do feel that you need salt in order to taste your food, then look at your zinc levels, which may be low. Zinc is involved in the optimum functioning of the taste buds. See p. 99 for more information about zinc levels.
Smoothies	I do not like tofu	The aim of the tofu is to provide some protein at breakfast or snacktime. If you wanted to, you could put in a tiny piece of tofu, and use unsweetened soya milk, which contains a little protein itself. Use protein powders if you prefer, but ensure that you follow instructions and also favour a sugar-free variety.

Eating out	I have to eat out frequently	You can still eat well if you have to eat out. Page 129 gives examples of how to eat in various different types of restaurants. Apply these principles whenever you can.
Snacking	I am too busy to shop every day for snacks	If you really have no time at all, then take advantage of the weekends and ensure that you buy a few small bags of raw nuts or seeds, and a large bag of apples. Keep some at work, or in your briefcase or rucksack, so that you have something easy to eat and accessible with you.
Cooking	I cannot cook or do not enjoy it	Cooking can be very easy but requires a little application. If you rely solely on shop-bought food you may not fully benefit from all that food has to offer. It is worth spending a small amount of time and a little effort in preparing as much of your own food as possible. After all, even sardines on toast is a balanced meal that requires very little preparation.
Detoxification	I have felt unwell during similar programmes	Minor headaches, or perhaps some fatigue or skin irritation, are not uncommon during such programmes. However, go at your own pace and if you feel unable to continue then stop the detoxification process and start again at another time. Remember that this process does not suit everyone, and you could consider undertaking a programme at another time under the supervision of a health professional.
Weight management	Can I stick to this for longer than one week?	The weight management programme has been designed to be followed for a period of one week. If you feel that you need to lose more weight, then remember that weight loss follows good health and by making good health your aim you could also lose some weight as well. Work with a qualified nutrition consultant to lose weight, rather than following any fad diets that might cause long-term problems in exchange for short-term weight loss.

afterword

Modern life has long overtaken many of our body's natural inbuilt abilities to cope, and life in the city can simply compound this. Stress affects almost every aspect of the body's functions, yet I believe we can do many things to minimize its potential to cause damage.

The toxins and pollution levels that are part of city life may all be within the limits that authorities deem to be safe. However, the cumulative effect of these chemicals can affect our health, either directly or indirectly. Allergies and intolerances have increased so much that once-rare food allergies are now becoming commonplace – I see many clients in my London practice who are manifesting symptoms of sensitivities to seemingly innocuous foods, and it is my personal belief that pollution and chemicals play a role in this increase. Furthermore, I believe that such substances will in the future be found to be involved in the rising incidence of many cancers.

Life is a series of choices, and while there is no correct way to live your life, I believe that what you eat plays a profound role. Choosing to benefit from the multitude of antioxidant and life-enhancing qualities of food can only serve to promote good health.

An absence of illness is not health – true health should involve vitality and energy – and changes to what we eat can help us both feel and function better, and enjoy all that city life has to offer. Taking responsibility for our own health is preferable to hoping that we will not be struck by illness. There are no guarantees, but the odds can be improved in our favour.

I hope that the information and suggestions in this book will appeal to as many readers as possible. They are all based on my clinical experience as a nutritional consultant and on personal experience of living in a large city. I encourage everyone to make positive choices: eating for vitality, good health and energy, leaving you in better shape to enjoy all that city life has to offer.

index

UK Organizations

British Diabetic Association
10 Queen Anne Street
London W1M 0BD
tel. 020 7323 1531

British Heart Foundation
14 Fitzhardings Street
London W1H 4DH
tel. 020 7935 0185

British Nutrition Foundation
52–54 High Holborn
London WC1V 6RQ
tel. 020 7404 6504

British Society for Mercury Free Dentistry
225 Old Brompton Road
London SW5 0EA
tel. 020 7373 3655

Coeliac Society
P.O. Box 220
High Wycombe
Buckinghamshire HP11 2HY
tel. 01494 437 278

Coronary Prevention Group
Suite 5/4
Plantation House
31/35 Fenchurch Street
London EC3M 3NN
tel. 020 7626 4844

Eating Disorders Association
Sackville Place
44 Magdalen Street
Norwich NR3 1JU
tel. 01603 621 414

Foresight
28 The Paddock
Godalming, Surrey GU7 1XD
tel. 01483 427 839

The Institute for Optimum Nutrition
Blades Court
Deodar Road
London, SW15 2NU
tel. 020 8877 9993

National Asthma Campaign
300 Upper Street
London N1
tel. 0345 010 203

National Eczema Society
Tavistock House
Tavistock Square
London WC1H 9SR
tel. 020 7388 4907

Society for the Promotion of Nutritional Therapy
P.O. Box 47
Heathfield
East Sussex
tel. 01825 872 921

The Soil Association
86 Colston Street
Bristol BS1 5BB
tel. 0117 929 0661

Vegetarian Society
Parkdale
Dunham Road
Altrincham
Cheshire WA14 4QG
tel. 0161 925 2000

World Cancer Research Fund
11–12 Buckingham Gate
London SW1E 6LB
tel. 020 7343 4200

US Organizations

American Association of World Health
1129–2012 st, NW, ste. 400
Washington DC 20036 3403

National Institute of Nutritional Education
1010 s. Jolier St
Aurora, CO 80012
tel. 800 530 8079

American Cancer Society
1599 Clifton Road
Atlanta
GA 30329
Tel. 800 - ACS-2345

American Heart Association
7272 Greenville Avenue
Dallas TX 75231
tel. 214 373 6300

American Diabetes Association
1660 Duke Street
Alexandria
VA 22314
tel. 800 232 3472

Crohn's and Colitis Foundation of America
386 Park Avenue
New York
NY 10016-8804
tel. 800 343 3637

Food Allergy Network
4744 Holly Avenue
Fairfax VA 22030-5647
tel. 703 691 3179

Lupus Foundation of America
4 Research Place
Rockville
MD 20850-3226
tel. 800 558 0121

Multiple Sclerosis Foundation
6350 North Andrews Avenue
Fort Lauderdale
FL 33309
tel. 800 441 7055

American Celiac Society
58 Musano Court
West Orange
NJ 07052
tel. 201 325 8837